total
stretch

total
stretch

roscoe nash

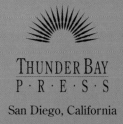

THUNDER BAY
P·R·E·S·S

San Diego, California

Thunder Bay Press

An imprint of the Advantage Publishers Group

5880 Oberlin Drive, San Diego, CA 92121-4794

www.thunderbaybooks.com

Copyright © MQ Publications 2003

Text copyright © Roscoe Nash 2003

Picture copyright © Corbis pages 8–9, 22–23, 128–129, 174–175

SERIES EDITOR: Kate John, MQ Publications

EDITORIAL DIRECTOR: Ljiljana Baird, MQ Publications

PHOTOGRAPHY BY Chris Perrett

DESIGN BY Balley Design Associates

ILLUSTRATION BY gerardgraphics.co.uk

ISBN 1-57145-804-2

Library of Congress Cataloging-in-Publication Data available upon request.

Printed in China

1 2 3 4 5 07 06 05 04 03

contents

the benefits of stretching

Stretching should become a regular routine for everyone, not just for professional athletes who already understand the benefits associated with performing a sequence of stretches. Some of these benefits are physically apparent, such as a greater range of movement, while others can't be seen, but are felt from within, such as an increased feeling of relaxation and general well-being. Stretching can become an unobtrusive and enjoyable part of your daily routine. You will soon find yourself doing it naturally and reaping the benefits permanently.

This book encompasses all the essential information on stretching. Parts One and Two focus on how to regulate your own personal stretching assessment and explain the physiology of stretching, in particular how it can alleviate health problems and improve mobility. A directory of core stretches makes up Part Three; these are presented according to each part of the body, from hamstrings to shoulders and from hips to abdominals. Part Four includes dynamic stretches and stretch programs suited to specific sporting activities, from playing tennis to swimming or practicing martial arts. Part Five shows how stretching can be incorporated into our daily routine; special routines are presented for office and manual work, and advice is given on back care and how to stretch while traveling.

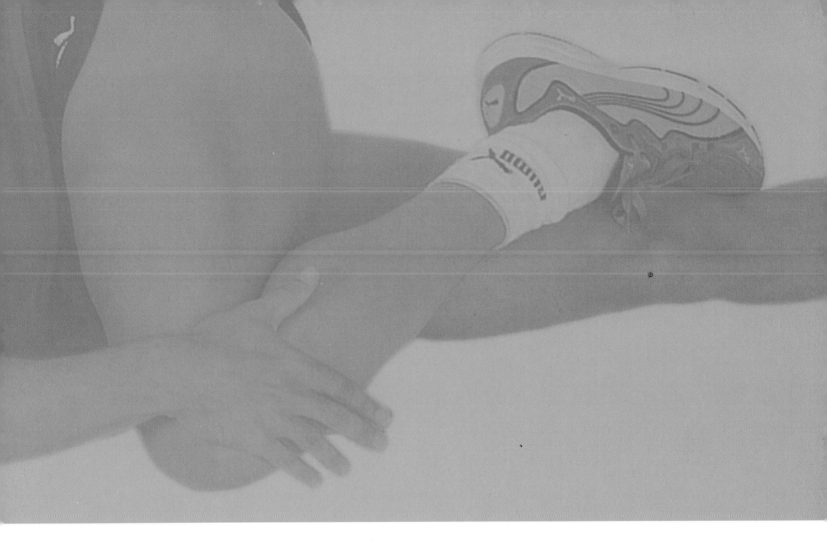

breathing and stretching

Breathing correctly is integral to achieving the most out of each individual stretch. By understanding how to control your breathing, you will learn how to extend further into a stretch gradually and safely. While you're stretching, breathing needs to be performed in one of two ways, depending on whether you're warming up or cooling down.

Your rate of breathing will naturally increase as your body exhales carbon dioxide from your lungs while taking in oxygen. Breathing deeply through your nose will help warm the air going into the lungs, while blowing air out through your mouth will help prepare the body for physical exercise. Adopt this method while stretching, increasing the tension on the stretch while exhaling. During the cool-down phase of exercise or while developing your stretches, your breathing should again be in via the nostrils and out via the mouth; however, you should gradually reduce your breathing rate by taking deeper breaths to fill the lungs, while slowly exhaling the air out. Breathing in brings new energy in the form of oxygen; breathing out relieves tension in the muscles and removes waste products.

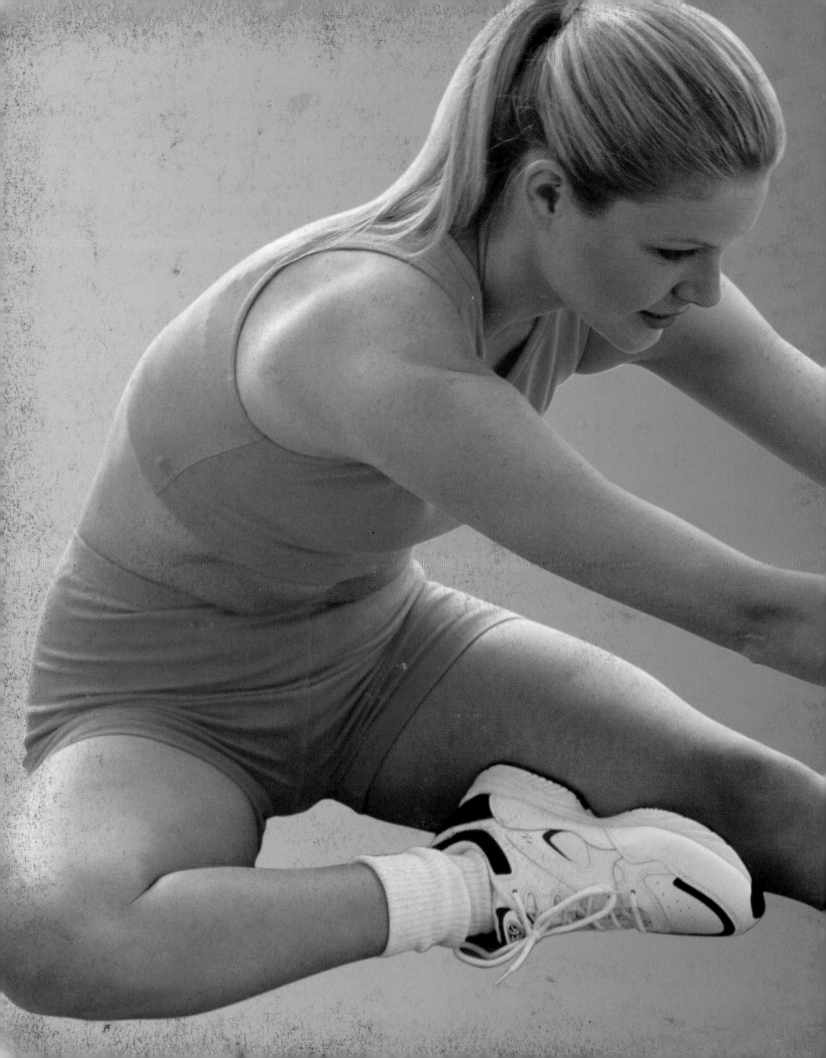

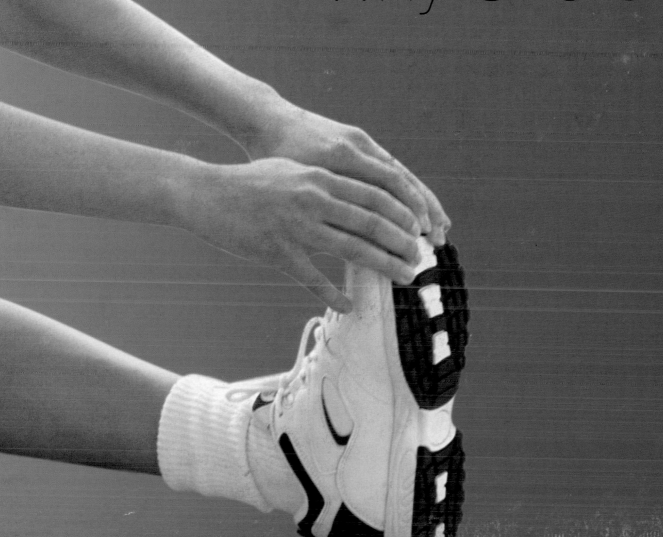

part 1

why stretch?

personal physical assessments

resting heart rate

The best time to take your resting heart rate is when you first wake up in the morning. If you take recordings over three days to find an average, you will get a more accurate reading. For example, readings taken on three consecutive mornings might be 75 bpm (beats per minute), 72 bpm, and 72 bpm. The average is then calculated by taking the total number of beats and dividing it by the number of mornings tested.

Answer: 75 + 72 + 72 = 219   219 ÷ 3 = 73 bpm

To take your heart rate, place two fingers on either your inside wrist (radial artery) or neck (carotid artery). Avoiding pressing too hard, count the number of beats during a minute. Perform this simple test over the next three days and then after one month, three months, and six months.

	date	bpm
day 1		
day 2		
day 3		
		average bpm
one month		
three months		
six months		

body awareness

Stretching enables you to become more aware of your body. Try this simple test, first using the index finger of your writing hand, then the index of your weaker hand. With your eyes closed, choose a number of precise points around your body and slowly place the index finger onto each point in turn. Score the test yourself by putting a check in the box if you place your finger onto the body point, or an X if you miss. Avoid choosing your eyes as one of these points (in case you poke yourself by mistake), and don't select moles, scars, or tattoos, as these will have no sensory paths to them, and as such, you will be working purely on memory.

	date	right hand	left hand
nose			
forehead			
opposite thumb			
opposite little finger			
left ankle			
right ankle			
belly button			
left ear			
right ear			

Use the different boxes for the results of each index finger, so you can see the difference between the left and right sides of your body.

flexibility test

The hamstring muscles (located at the back of the upper leg) are tight in most people, especially in men and soccer players.

Sit on the floor with shoes removed and place the soles of your feet flat against a wall. Take your fingers toward the wall without bouncing or forcing your body into the stretch. Make sure that the movement is controlled and doesn't cause pain.

Keeping your back and legs straight, bend at the lower back/waist. Focus on trying to touch the wall with the tips of your fingers. You may need to do this test with a partner so that he/she can use a ruler to measure how far away you are from the wall.

If you can touch the wall comfortably with your fingers, then you may want to try sliding your fingers along a coffee table, again keeping your legs and back straight. For accurate progression results, use the same table each time you try this test.

The distance you measure will either be the distance away from the wall in the first method or the distance across the table in the second method. For the table method, you may want to push an object, such as a pencil, to make the measuring easier.

date	distance

why warm up?

Imagine your muscles to be like a piece of clay. When you first pick up the clay, you will find that it is dry and hard. You can bend it into the shape you want, but will soon find that it splits and eventually breaks in two. After adding a little water and some warmth from rolling the clay in your hands, the same nonpliable piece of clay quickly becomes soft and pliable and you are able to mold it into a whole array of shapes.

The same can be said for your muscles. When cold, they can be stretched, but muscle receptors restrict you from overstretching them to prevent muscle damage. This means that you cannot achieve a full stretch unless the muscle is warmed up properly. When you are placing high levels of stress upon the muscle (i.e., when exercising), it is important that the muscle be warmed up so that you can perform the exercise without becoming injured.

As with clay, in order to achieve a greater level of stretch within the muscle, spend time warming up. A gradual increase in the heart rate will enable the warmth of the blood, passing more and more rapidly through the muscle to steadily improve the muscle's pliability.

Look at your warm-up as a sequence of logical events that will give you the following benefits:

- A reduced risk of injury to the joints, muscles, and tendons
- A reduction in muscular soreness and tension
- An increase in heart rate, blood flow, body temperature, nerve impulses, metabolic rate, and oxygen utilization
- Greater body awareness and mental alertness
- Improved range of motion and enhanced physical ability
- Sport-specific stretching and the ability to focus on the task ahead

how to warm up

The warm-up is one of the key elements in a successful stretching program, and you should allocate an adequate amount of time within your workout or stretching routine to enable your muscles to become adequately warm. Muscles can only achieve maximum performance when all their blood vessels are dilated, enabling sufficient blood flow. At rest, muscles only use 15–20 percent of blood flow, compared to 70 percent, or more, after only ten minutes of activity.

The warm-up can be passive, using an outside source such as a hot shower, hot tub, massage, sauna, or extra clothing. Alternatively, it can be active, using body movement to generate warmth. During the active phase, athletes should concentrate on imitating the movements that they will be performing when in full flow, for example, controlled punching prior to actually boxing or taking a kick-boxing class.

Runners tend to stretch their cold muscles before going for a run, and as such have little or no benefit from the time they spend stretching. Greater results would be achieved if stretching were carried out after ten minutes of fast walking/slow jogging.

Because the passive method works on warming up the superficial outer layer of the body (i.e., the skin), we actually get the feeling of warmth. This method is not as effective as an active warm-up, because, with the exception of massage, there is no major increase in the blood flow through the muscles, and, as such, it is only really suitable as a warm up before an activity.

The best way to warm up is to combine both methods where possible. If you are just performing a stretching program, consider spending time in a warm bath first to help raise your body temperature. When you come out of the bath, dress in warm clothing that allows you to perform the stretches without restrictions. After your bath, spend a minimum of five minutes performing active movements prior to any actual stretching.

Using the larger muscle groups, such as the quadriceps (upper thighs) and the gluteal muscles (buttocks), is the most effective way to relocate your warming blood from areas such as the digestive system to the muscles.

The length of time you spend warming up will vary depending upon your age, fitness level, and the room temperature. You should be developing a light sweat, a feeling of general looseness, and a greater range of mobility prior to going into the stretch phase.

You need to stay warm throughout your stretching, so you should quickly dry any sweat away. Ideally your hair should not be wet from your shower. If possible, the room temperature should be increased slightly or an extra layer of nonrestrictive clothing worn. If you start to feel cold or your range of movement throughout the stretch is not what you normally perform, warm up your body again and then continue with your stretching.

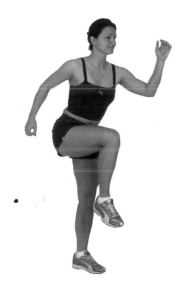

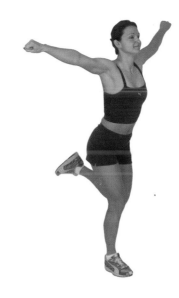

❶ March on the spot, gradually taking your knees a little higher, while at the same time working your arms and doing the finger, wrist, and elbow mobility exercises. Two minutes.

❷ Follow this by taking one leg behind you, alternately, while raising both your arms out to the side (no higher than shoulder level). One minute.

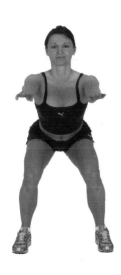

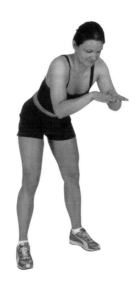

❸ Do some simple squats – holding your arms at just below shoulder level, take your hands to the front as you squat down and then your elbows to the rear as you come up to standing. Thirty seconds.

❹ Simulate a swimming action, arms only—front crawl, backstroke, butterfly, breaststroke. Fifteen seconds each movement.

A very simple active warm-up can consist of the following routine. You may already have your own routine or suitable aerobic video that you prefer to use. Repeat the above once more or until you feel warm.

mobility—lubricating your joints

Just like the engine in a car has oil to prevent the damage of metal rubbing against metal, the body has its own lubricating fluid, synovial fluid, which helps prevent wear and tear on the joint surfaces from bones rubbing against each other. When we wake up in the morning, this synovial fluid has drained back into its own reservoir around the joint (synovial membrane)—just like the oil within the car engine, which sinks to the bottom. When we wake up or become active after long periods of inactivity, we should perform the following sequence to "lubricate" the body.

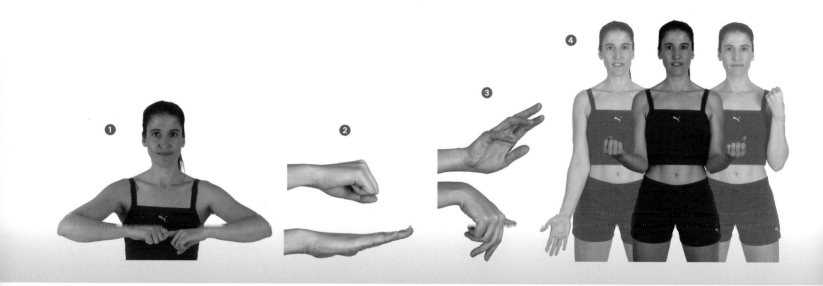

❶ finger pull

Grasp each finger at the base between the index and middle finger of the opposite hand. Keeping the finger straight, slowly pull on each finger two to three times with mild pressure.

❷ fingers and knuckles

Simply clench your fist and flick out your fingers for three seconds, then gradually increase the speed so that you are clenching and flicking your fingers twice in a single second. Perform this action for ten seconds, working both hands.

❸ wrists

Rotate your wrists clockwise and then counterclockwise in a slow, controlled motion, followed by simple flexion and extension of the wrists, with your fingers pointing straight out.

❹ elbows

Begin with controlled flexion and extension of the arm, bending at the elbow joint with your arms tucked into your side. As you perform this action, turn the palms of your hands toward and then away from the body in order to create a slight twisting action at the elbow joint.

❺ shoulders

Raise your shoulders slowly upward toward your ears in small movements, then allow your shoulders to relax downward naturally. Breathe in through your nose as you raise your shoulders, exhaling the air from your lungs in the downward phase. Gradually make the movements larger and then switch to a circular motion of the shoulder joint, taking the shoulder in backward and forward circles. You may want to work the

The sequence of movements involved for mobility is similar to those that are performed throughout your normal day, so if time is a major factor, you may wish to begin with your warm-up, which will also aid in lubricating your joints. Once you are confident with each individual mobility exercise, you may wish to combine the exercises into your own routine, for example, working the fingers, wrists, and elbows all at the same time.

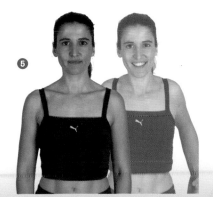
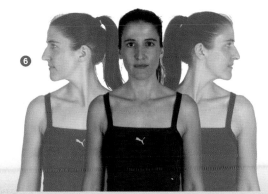
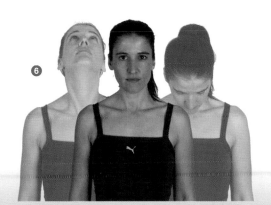

shoulders together or each separately. Whichever you choose, work for a minimum of thirty seconds on each side, as your shoulders are generally the first area of the body to suffer when you are under any stress.

❻ neck

Look over one shoulder, then slowly turn your head to look over the other shoulder in an overemphasized "no" motion. Repeat this five to ten times each side, taking two seconds for each movement. After the "no" movement, perform a "yes" nodding action, taking your head downward, then upward, repeating five to ten times and holding each movement for two seconds. Next gently tilt your head toward your shoulders. Do not force this movement—as you start, gently let your head relax down toward your shoulder. Repeat five times each side,

making each movement last five seconds. (Note: Stop immediately if you experience any feeling of dizziness and do not repeat.) You can finish by rotating the head in a clockwise and counterclockwise motion. Focus on simulating a spiral effect, starting with small movements and working out to gradually larger movements, keeping the action under control at all times. Spend only a short time doing this exercise, as it can irritate the tiny neck joints. Think about keeping your neck "long" throughout (therefore avoiding taking your head back too far). If you have a very stiff or sore neck, it is best to avoid this exercise altogether.

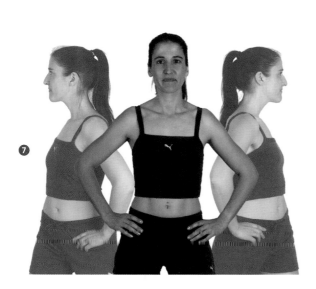

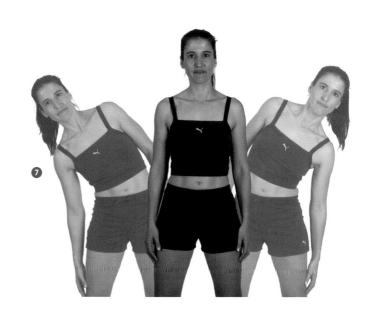

❼ trunk/waist

Keeping your hands on your waist, make small, twisting movements from your waist to take one elbow forward and the other one back. Follow this by sliding each hand downward on your leg toward your knees. Throughout both actions, you should be standing with your feet shoulder width apart and your pelvis facing forward. Keep the motion under control and avoid swinging or bouncing. Remember that you are only warming up the joints.

❽ hips

Depending upon your balance, you may want to hold onto a chair for support. In a controlled motion, extend one leg forward, then directly behind in small movements, keeping the leg straight. Repeat three to five times. Placing your other leg on a raised platform will enable you to perform these routines without the foot of the working leg making contact with the floor. Take the same leg out to the side of the body (this is called "abduction"), again in small movements. Repeat three to five times. Finally, perform small, circular motions with the leg, taking the leg from the center outward, first in a forward and then in a backward direction, always controlling the movement of the leg. After you have performed these three simple movements, you can repeat the complete process again, but this time make the movements slightly larger. If you find that standing on the same leg is uncomfortable, you should change legs frequently, ideally before any discomfort is felt. You may find it more comfortable having a slight bend (soft knees) in the leg you are not working.

❾ ankles/toes

Perform the same sequence for the ankles as for the wrist, using circular motions in both directions, followed by flexion and extension of the foot. After this, place your heels on the ground and raise your toes off the floor. Concentrate on curling up and relaxing your toes.

❿ knees

Again holding onto a chair for support, if you choose, flex the leg to bring your foot behind you. Repeat this action on both legs ten to fifteen times in a smooth, controlled motion. Follow this action on both legs by performing a circular motion of the foot from the knee joint in both clockwise and counterclockwise directions, five to ten times. You may find it easier to perform this and the ankle and toe exercises while seated on a chair.

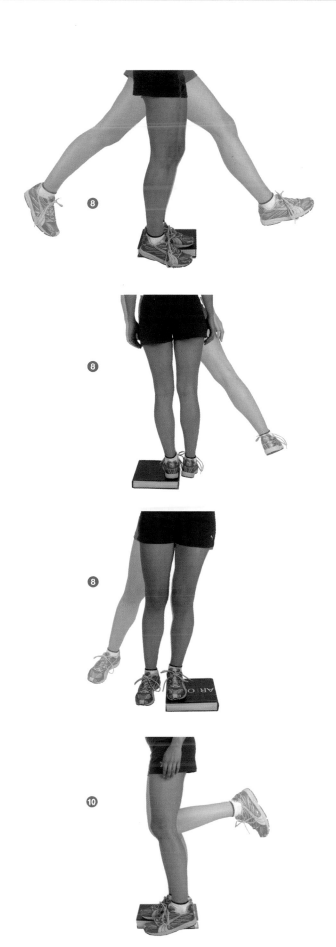

finding the right stretching technique

There are numerous methods of stretching, each with their own pros and cons. For beginners, however, the most common and safest form would be static stretching.

static stretching This method involves holding a stretch at a point where the muscle is under full stretch. It is easy to learn and considered one of the safest methods, while still giving a good stretch to the muscle if carried out after a suitable warm-up. Its main disadvantage is for general activity, in that while stretching, the body's muscles are getting cold. For some individuals this may mean that their muscles have not been specifically placed under the amount of exertion that they are used to in their regular activity.

isometric stretching Another form of static stretching comprising the tension of a muscle while in its isometric phase (fixed point of contraction, normally at the halfway point of its range of movement). An example would be pushing against a wall to stretch the calf muscle. Isometric stretching is not recommended for children or adolescents, as their bones are still growing and this method places pressure on the tendons.

PNF stretching (proprioceptive neuromuscular facilitation) This method of stretching can produce excellent, rapid results because of its technique in using isometric contraction of the muscle before the stretch is carried out. PNF is normally done with the assistance of a partner, as good communication between both people is essential in order to achieve optimum results and avoid injury.

ballistic stretching This is a method of stretching that is being slowly eliminated due to numerous studies showing that uncontrolled bouncing movements trigger the stretch reflex (a part of the muscle that increases muscular tension to avoid any tearing within the muscle). It is still used by many martial artists and dancers, due to the explosive actions these people perform. This method does not allow the muscle to relax or stretch, it is simply forced into the lengthening procedure, for example, when standing with legs straight and bending at the waist to touch the floor with your fingers.

dynamic stretching Unlike ballistic stretching, dynamic stretching uses the movement in a controlled motion that is ideally simulated to that of the chosen activity, for example, a swimmer does swimming motions on dry land. Dynamic stretching is a good method of preparing the body for high-level activities, but care should be taken to avoid exerting yourself too much as you begin the motions. This type of stretching is best performed after a thorough warm-up.

passive (or relaxed) stretching Passive stretching is when you hold a relaxed position with your body—either on your own, with a partner, or using a specific piece of equipment—and make no active contribution to the stretch. A good example is lying on your back with your legs against a wall and allowing gravity to increase the stretch. Passive stretching is excellent for tight muscles or for areas that are difficult to stretch because the muscles are too weak to activate the stretch for themselves.

active stretching Generally classed into three groups—free active, active assisted, and resisted. Active stretching increases active flexibility and strengthens the agonistic muscles (agonistic relates to the muscle being contracted), as a free active stretch is one where your adopted position is held only by the main agonist muscle groups. For example, holding your leg straight to the left while seated uses the quadriceps (agonists) to relax the hamstrings (antagonists). Antagonistic relates to the muscle that is relaxed. Active assisted stretches will make use of either a partner or a towel to increase the range within the stretch. This method is used a lot in yoga and is suitable for those who have weak agonist muscles. Resistive active stretching makes use of resistance being applied to the stretch while contracting the muscle.

muscle energy technique This technique is very useful where muscle tone is so tight (hypertonic) that it is almost impossible to stretch without risking injury. It is also useful for stretching difficult muscle groups, such as the biceps, for example—either on your own or with the help of a partner. It takes advantage of a state of muscle function, i.e., fatigue mode, to make stretching easier. You can use this technique on very tight neck muscles, for example. Resting your elbow on a tabletop or similar surface, support your head under the chin with the hand of the same arm. Next turn your head to one side, while resisting the movement with the supporting hand. Hold the movement to the count of forty and then repeat, with hardly any break for rest, at least five times. Wait ten seconds and then make the movement again, this time with no resistance, and see how much further you can go as you stretch out muscles that are temporarily fatigued.

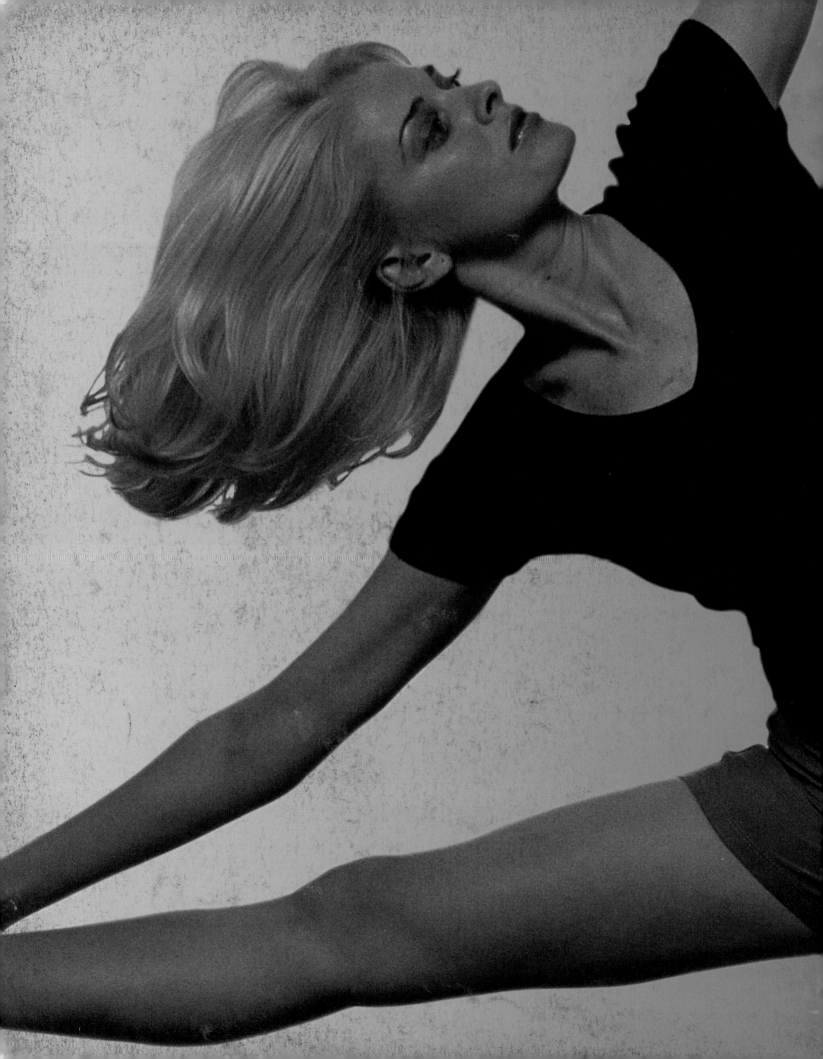

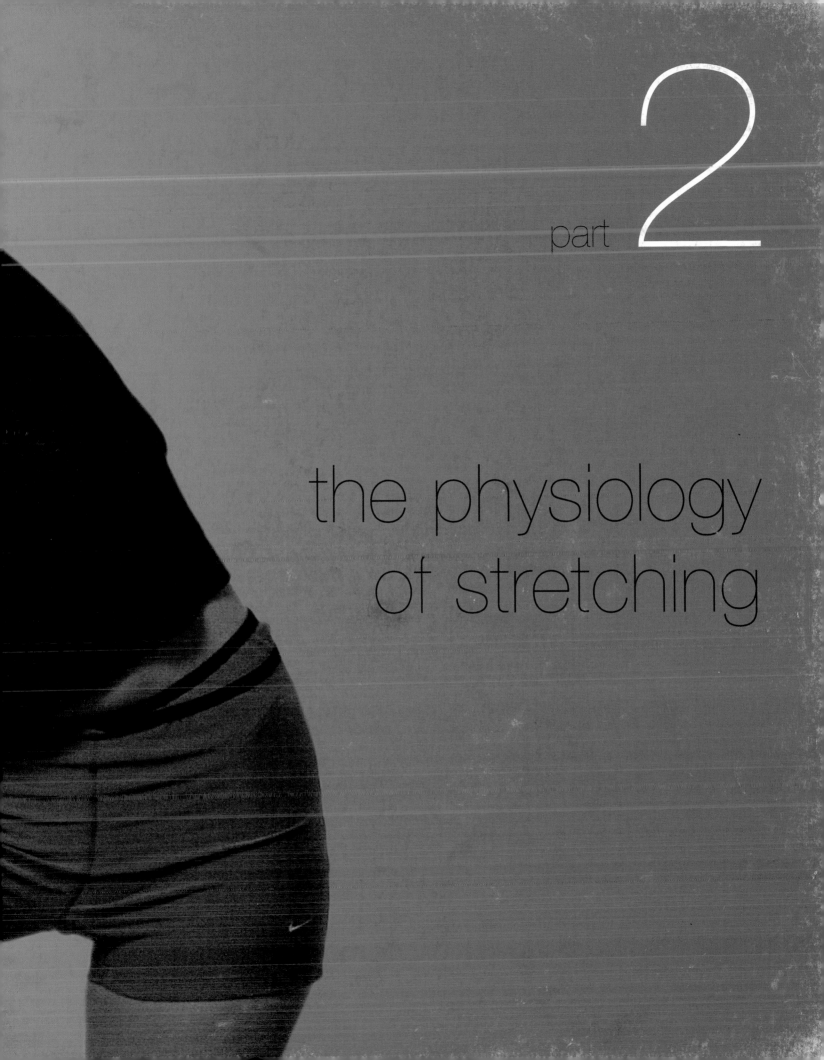

the physiology
of stretching

the importance of the role of the musculoskeletal system

When we talk about stretching the body, we are describing stretching a system known as the musculoskeletal system. This system includes the bones of the skeleton, along with the ligaments and the muscles and their tendons, which help to move and support these bones.

The musculoskeletal system has developed primarily for the purpose of locomotion or movement. It also provides an excellent supporting/protective system to the vulnerable internal organs, whose main role is to provide the musculoskeletal system with nourishment, stimulation, and purification. Many people consider the nervous system, including the brain, and the circulatory system, including the heart, to be the most important systems. It goes without saying that if the heart stops and the brain ceases to function, the body dies. However, without the body being able to move and generate energy and heat, search for food, help circulate the blood and lymph, expand the rib cage in order to breathe, and perform numerous evasive movements in order to protect itself, it would not be able to exist and function naturally. Therefore, it would be quite reasonable to state that the musculoskeletal system is the most important system. By accepting its importance, we must also recognize that the need to maintain it in top condition should be paramount. If this is difficult to understand and accept, consider the plights of people who suffer from advanced muscular dystrophy, or are totally paralyzed. Gradually their organs fail, their lungs cannot function properly, or unaided, due to weakness in the respiratory muscles, and the lack of posture causes a stasis in both the lungs and the circulation, normally resulting in severe infections and eventual death.

the components of the musculoskeletal system

There are three main components to this intricate system, all working in conjunction with each other and all having some effect on the system as a whole. The first component is the skeleton.

skeleton

The skeleton consists of numerous bones, whose shape and structure reflects their role and which are brought into contact with each other to make a joint. This gives rise to a structure made of a very solid, strong material, which is able to articulate. The outer layers of the bones consist of a hard, dense material, while the centers are made of a spongy cortex that makes the bones lighter, otherwise we would not be able to move our own weight! This cortex also provides a medium for the rich network of blood vessels to penetrate through the bones, providing nourishment and transporting away

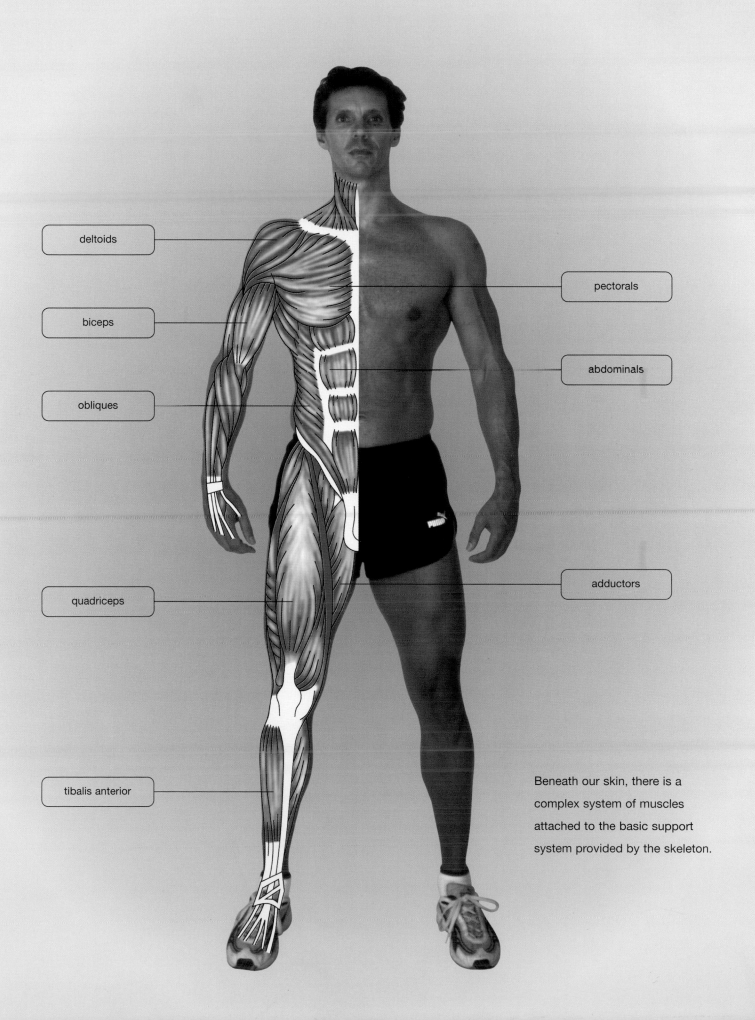

deltoids

pectorals

biceps

abdominals

obliques

quadriceps

adductors

tibalis anterior

Beneath our skin, there is a complex system of muscles attached to the basic support system provided by the skeleton.

the new red blood cells that are manufactured in some bones. The ends of all articulating bones are covered in a cartilaginous surface (hyaline), which helps to protect the bones against the wear and tear caused by continual movement and friction, and allows the bones to glide over, or against, each other. Articulating joints are called synovial joints, because, as well as the ends of the bones being covered with cartilage, the whole joint is encased in a capsule, a bit like a sleeve/tube enveloping both ends together. Lining this capsule is a membrane called the synovial membrane, which produces a fluid (synovial fluid) that lubricates the surfaces.

ligaments

To keep these joints aligned properly with one another is our second component, the ligaments. These are straplike structures consisting of dense, fibrous tissue, which are positioned in such a way as to allow movement, but also to restrict the range of movement to within a safe level to prevent damage to adjacent tissues and structures. Ligaments also assist in support. Ligaments are normally positioned around the joint and outside of the joint capsule (extracapsular).

example

If you have ever strained your ankle or knee, you will find this easy to understand. The ligaments that support those two areas allow flexion, extension, and some degree of rotation. In the case of the knee, there are two important extra ligaments called cruciates (because they cross over each other). These are located inside the joint capsule (intracapsular) and limit the forward/backward shift of the femur (thigh bone) on the tibia (leg bone). Damage to any of these ligaments, as a result of injury and trauma, can give rise to sudden misalignment of the bones, pain and swelling in the joint itself, and instability, which frequently leads to subsequent recurrence of the same injury. Treatment is normally based on restabilizing the joint with some form of strapping, and because this normally works well, demonstrates the importance of the role of the ligaments in both posture and joint stability. It is also important in a newly strained joint that you reduce the swelling that usually occurs as a result of inflammation. If the swelling, which is a buildup of fluid in the tissues, is allowed to persist, it will cause some structures to be stretched, especially unaffected ligaments, thus aggravating the problem. Reducing the inflammation by locally applied cold compresses and anti-inflammatory gel will greatly assist the overall healing process. Homeopathic remedies can also be very beneficial. All of these remedies are most effective if initiated immediately after the injury occurs.

muscles

Our third component is the muscles—probably the most complex yet versatile group of the three. Without muscles there can be no movement. Each muscle has a main part, or belly, and two ends called tendons. Muscles are normally firmly attached on the two bones on either side of a joint via their tendons, and when the belly contracts, it shortens. In doing so, the tendons pull against their attachment on the bones, shortening the distance between the two bones and causing a movement at the joint. Skeletal muscles can also contract to cause other types of movement not involving joints, e.g., facial muscles contract to produce a smile; the diaphragm contracts, causing the lungs to inflate. Skeletal muscle is made up of thousands of muscle fibers all joined together in bundles and separated by layers of fibrous connective tissue. Many of the layers of fibrous tissue extend the whole length of the muscle and end as part of the tendon that will attach to the surface of the bone. This continuity helps to provide the strength to the muscle structure. The shape of a muscle and the size, shape, and direction of the muscle fibers can vary greatly between one muscle and the next, as they are all are designed to fulfill a particular role. The saying "structure is related to function" is most applicable here. Muscle and bone are two completely different tissues, therefore they need a third substance to help bond them together, just like wood and glass need putty. This third tissue, periosteum, is an outer covering to the bone, which is fibrous, allowing the fibers of the muscle tendon to blend with it and thus form an attachment between tendon and bone.

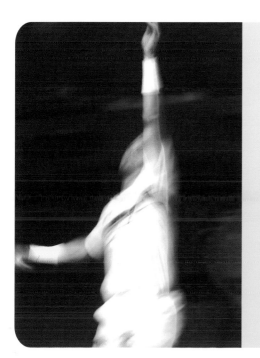

anyone for tennis? The condition known as tennis elbow arises as a result of too much tension being exerted by the tendon at its periosteal site, just above the elbow. The site at which the tendon attaches can be quite small in area, yet the pull on that area can be extremely high.

With persistently tight extensor forearm muscles, the continual pull by the extensor tendons can actually cause the beginning of a separation of the various fibrous layers of the periosteum. This leads to inflammatory changes taking place within the area, which in turn leads to further irritation of the muscle. Hence a vicious circle is set up. To treat this type of strain, you need to reduce both the tension within the muscle by rest and/or stretching, and reduce the inflammation locally with ice packs, anti-inflammatory gel, or, if necessary, a cortisone injection.

how do muscles work?

Skeletal muscle tissue is connected to both the nervous system and the circulatory system, and needs both in order to function.

the nerve supply

First, a muscle cannot initiate a contraction without a nerve impulse stimulating an electrical impulse at a site known as the neuromuscular junction. This simply translates as "no nerve impulse, no muscle activity," which is clearly demonstrated where nerves have been severed or damaged due to trauma and where paralysis occurs. Where each nerve cell sends an impulse to a muscle cell, a motor unit is formed. The number of muscle fibers supplied by that motor unit will determine the type of function of that particular muscle. If the motor unit is linked to just a few fibers (taking into account that this particular muscle may consist of thousands of motor unit/fiber components), a refined contractile movement of part of the muscle can be obtained, giving a more precise movement. This is seen in the muscles of the hands and face, for example. In muscles where one motor unit is linked to thousands of fibers, a more basic substantial contraction is involved, e.g., in the large, bulky muscles of the legs.

The stimulation by the nerve impulse releases two main chemical components—calcium and a high energy compound called adenosine triphosphate, or ATP. In simple terms the calcium switches on the muscle and the ATP provides the energy for the contraction activity to be performed (this chemical release activates extremely tiny filaments that make up the muscle fiber to slide across each other, causing a shortening of the muscle fiber, which results in a contraction). The withdrawal of calcium back into the cells switches off the muscle contraction and switches on muscle relaxation. The strength of the muscle contraction is influenced by many factors. These include the initial length of the muscle fibers, the metabolic state of the fiber, the number of motor units and fibers activated, and the load put on them.

the stretch receptors

The nervous system supplies muscles with the means to contract (motor), and the sensory system gives feedback (sensory) to the brain, telling it what is going on within the muscle and where. This sensory system includes specialized sensory (stretch) receptors, called muscle spindles, and Golgi tendon organs, which are capable of detecting the degree of stretch in both the muscle and its junction with the tendon, respectively. These receptors act as warning systems and will prevent the muscle from damage due to overstretching. As the muscle is stretched, the muscle spindles are stretched, and the stretch receptors are activated, sending a signal to the brain, which initiates a motor impulse to encourage contraction to occur, thus preventing any overstretching of the fibers. This feedback mechanism is called the reflex arc.

In summary, the motor nerve fibers instigate an impulse that leads to a contraction, which results in the stretching of other muscles. Stretching sends off a signal to the brain, which then leads to the stretched muscle contracting and regaining its shape/length, which is important in protecting it from injury. The signals that are sent from the muscle spindle to the brain are fired at a particular rate, which helps to clarify to the brain the exact degree of stretch, i.e., the change in length and the speed of change. In a slow, controlled stretch, it is possible to retrain these receptors to become accustomed to a new length, before they trigger off the impulse to contract to protect themselves.

Skeletal muscles almost always act in groups, and movements are produced by the coordinated action of several muscles. The way these groups work will vary depending on their role. Having stated that if a stretch occurs, an automatic signal will be activated to cause a contraction and end the stretch, it is necessary to add that this is not always so. There are some muscle groups that work in cooperation with each other as agonists and antagonists, e.g., the hamstrings and the quadriceps groups. As the agonists contract, the antagonists are forced to relax. If this did not happen you would never be able to bend your knee, as there would be an ongoing power struggle between the two sets of muscles. The muscles that actually cause the movement are referred to as the prime movers. Muscles that contract at the same time as the prime mover and help to stabilize a part of that movement are known as synergists. For example, in the calf, the gastrocnemius muscle is the prime mover and the soleus, located underneath the gastrocnemius, is the synergist.

below: Here you can see the skeletal muscle groups that cooperate to allow the elbow and knee joints to move in a coordinated action.

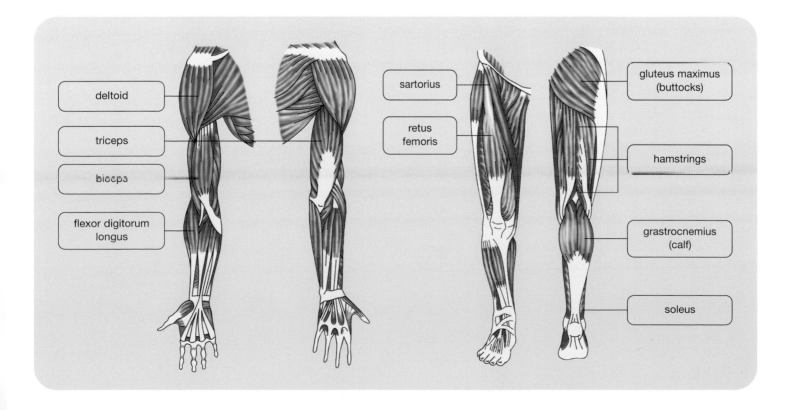

deltoid

triceps

biceps

flexor digitorum longus

sartorius

retus femoris

gluteus maximus (buttocks)

hamstrings

grastrocnemius (calf)

soleus

Continuous feedback occurs automatically between muscle tissue and the brain, via the nervous system. If damage or disease occurs to the peripheral nerve itself or at the neuromuscular junction, complete loss of tone can result. Causes can range from trauma or pressure, but also include disorders such as diabetes, multiple sclerosis, and the various forms of muscular dystrophy. Damage to the upper motor neuron within the brain usually results in disorders of increased tone and spasm.

the blood supply to the muscles

The circulatory system not only supplies blood by means of its arterial system, but also allows blood to drain from the tissues via its venous system. In the case of muscle tissue, both systems are equally important.

The arterial supply to the muscle is essential in providing the muscle with a continuously available source of calcium and the components needed to manufacture ATP within the cells. The venous drainage allows all the waste by-products of muscle activity to be taken away from the muscle itself. One of the main by-products is lactic acid, and a buildup of this within the muscle is what can cause what we commonly call a stitch.

Taking into account these facts should help you understand the overall concept of keeping the body supple and flexible, as the circulation, particularly the venous drainage element, requires rhythmic movement to encourage blood flow back toward the heart and lungs for purification. Extremely tight calf muscles can prevent this from happening satisfactorily. The regular rhythmic contractions of both the calf and buttock muscles combine to form a "pump" mechanism, which, in conjunction with a valve mechanism in the main veins of the lower limbs, encourages blood flow upward against gravity. People who sit all day or stand still in one place for long periods of time can compromise this mechanism. Typical symptoms of this are tired and achy feet and legs, and swollen feet and ankles. The ache directly results from the waste products being held too long within the muscle tissue.

posture and muscle tone

Gravity has a continual pull on the various parts of the body at all times. Our evolutionary development, ending with us standing upright on two legs, has meant extensive adaptation of our mechanism over the years. Posture has to be maintained using the minimum amount of energy, which is why people with poor posture suffer with tired, aching muscles. Any posture, whether it is sitting or standing, bending or stretching, is achieved by the combination and coordination of different muscle groups contracting and relaxing in order to achieve balance. If one or more groups are not able to take advantage of regular episodes of relaxation in between their role as contractors (perhaps because in doing so balance would be lost), then these groups will eventually fatigue, having used excessive energy to maintain their workload, and their tissue state would suffer. In order to consider good posture; look at yourself sideways in the mirror and ask yourself "Does more stick out the front than it does the back?" Sounds crazy? It shouldn't, because if your body is being encouraged to lean forward due to poor abdominal tone, excess weight, or slumped and rounded shoulders, what do you think is keeping you from falling flat on your face? The answer is overworked, tight, and tired back and calf muscles. This is why it is important to keep your weight down, maintain good abdominal tone, and help to keep those back muscles loose and relaxed. This is the reason that regular stretching of your back and lower limb muscles is really important. Statistics show that more days are lost at work from back strain than any other injury.

age-related problems and changes due to injury

Skeletal muscle undergos various methods of repair. In young, healthy adults with a steady supply of the components essential for these repairs, damaged tissue will be repaired as new, resulting in continuity of elastic muscle fibers. In older people, as fibers degenerate naturally or become damaged, they are not repaired with elastin-containing components, but are instead replaced with fibrous tissue, a process called fibrosis. This fibrous connective tissue may be relatively strong, but is unable to stretch as well as muscle, and because it contains no actual muscle fibers, cannot contract. In essence, a muscle can gradually become so fibrosed that the ratio of muscle fibers to connective tissue becomes so low that the muscle loses its ability to function as a muscle and weakness occurs. While this is an unfortunate part of the aging process, a similar situation can occur as a result of repeated injuries at the same site. This is often seen in soccer players, where the calf muscles can receive severe injuries from kicking. The tissues heal with fibrotic changes, which can lead to an inability to stretch the calf properly, and can subsequently lead to injuries occurring to other parts of the body as a result of an inability to move freely. Fibrotic tissue in the calves does not possess the same amount of elasticity and therefore cannot assist the calf pump mechanism. People who undergo surgery for repair to damaged tissue should begin stretching the area gently, yet persistently, to prevent connective tissue layers from sticking together as adhesions and giving the same long-term problems as fibrosed muscles.

   In summary, throughout our lives we should make a regular effort to maintain our body by stretching, keeping our joints supple, and getting our circulation moving.

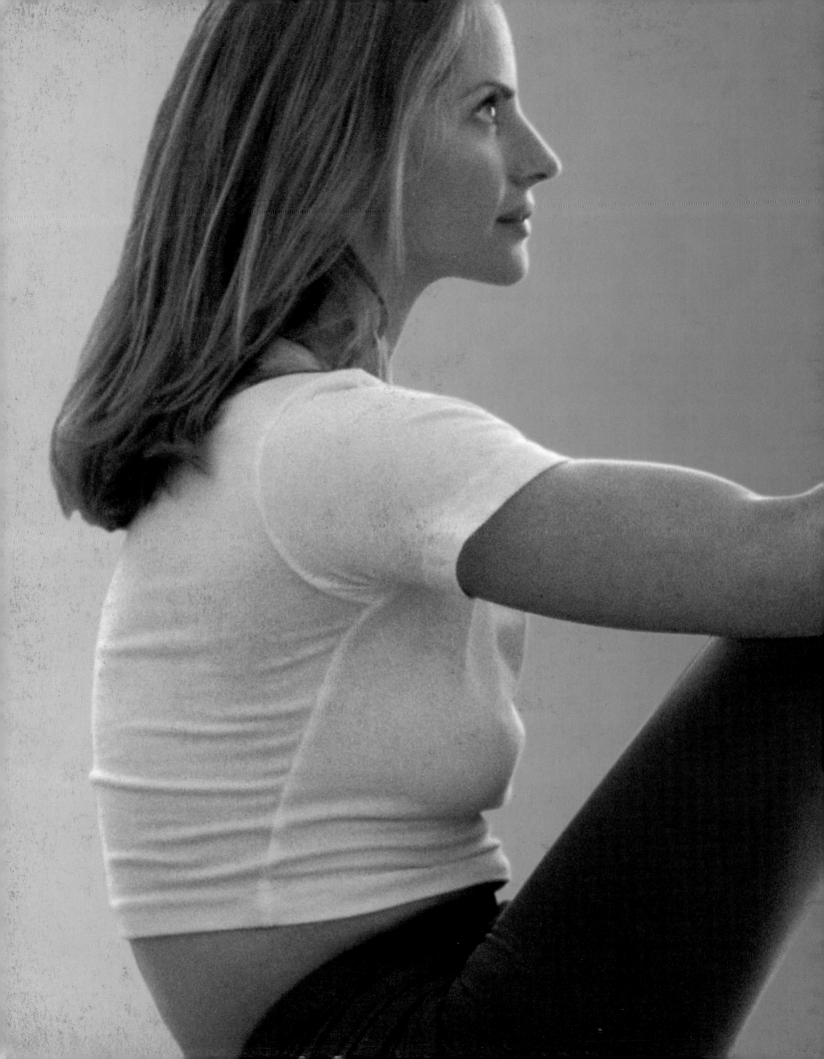

part 3

the stretches

the back

lower back **cat stretch**

easy

❶ Adopt a position on all fours, pointing your fingers forward and your toes behind.

❷ Start with a flat back and then drop your head downward, pushing your
shoulder blades upward and outward as you elevate your upper back.

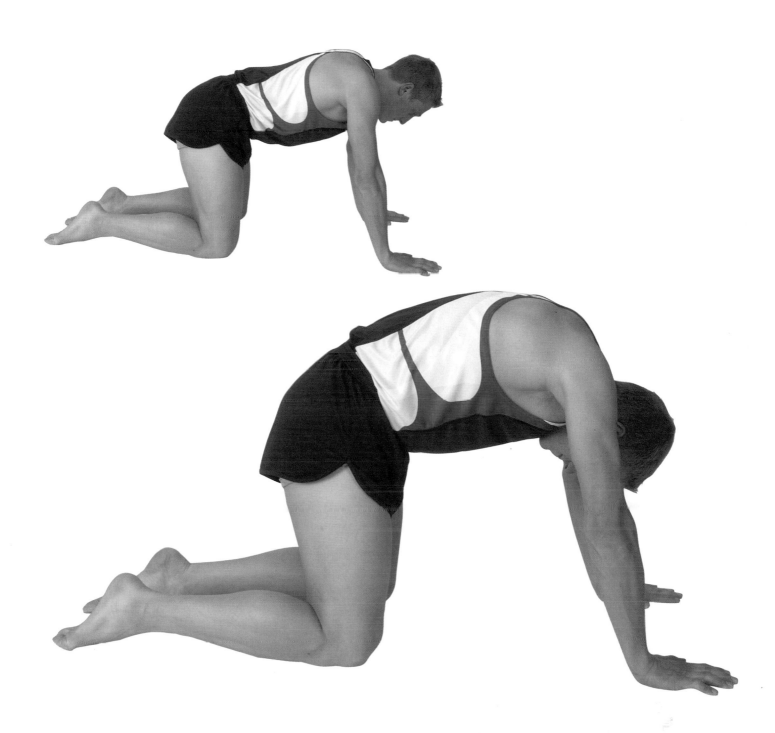

upper back **leg grab**

`easy`

❶ While seated, exhale, bending forward and hugging your thighs underneath with both arms.

❷ Keep your feet extended out as you pull your chest down onto your thighs, keeping both knees together.

❸ While in this position, you can also stretch your rhomboids by pulling your upper back away from your knees while still grasping your legs.

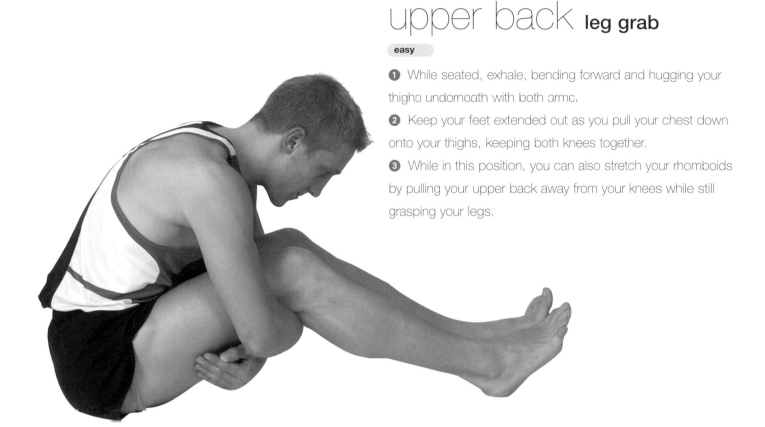

fetal position

`easy`

❶ Lie on your back, keeping your head on the floor.

❷ Slowly pull both legs into your chest and secure them there by wrapping your arms around the back of your knees.

❸ Exhale, pulling down on your legs while gradually lifting your buttocks off the floor.

❹ You can stretch your neck once you are in this position by slowly tilting your chin to your chest.

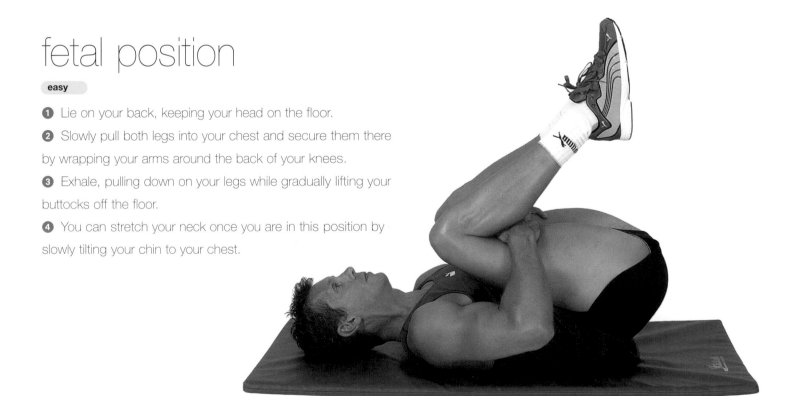

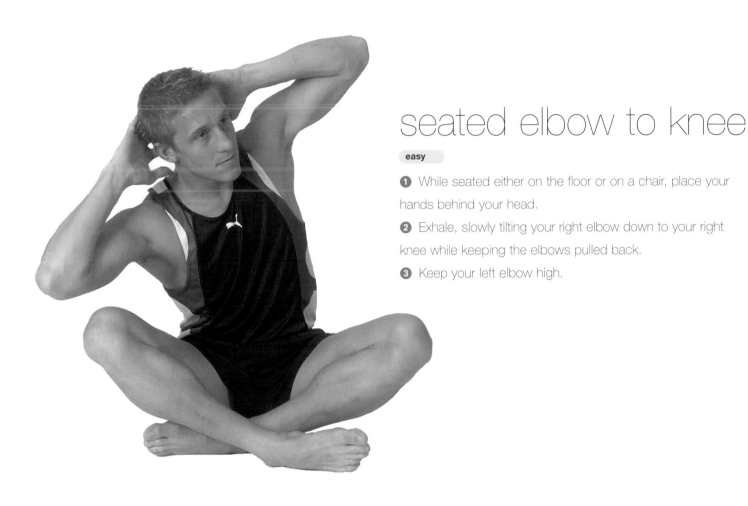

seated elbow to knee

easy

1 While seated either on the floor or on a chair, place your hands behind your head.

2 Exhale, slowly tilting your right elbow down to your right knee while keeping the elbows pulled back.

3 Keep your left elbow high.

pull and push

easy

1 Rest on your knees with your hands extended out to your front, grasping a secure object.

2 Exhale, gradually pushing your chest and abdomen downward to arch your spine.

3 Increase the stretch in your lower back by tilting your pelvis upward.

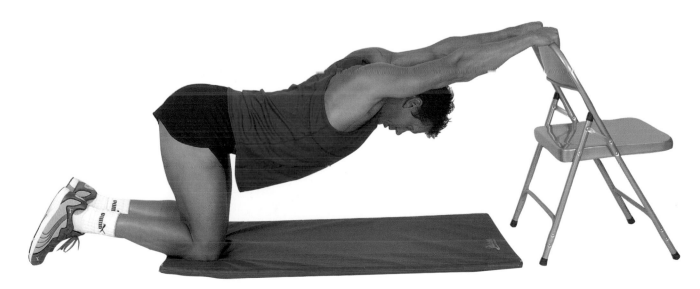

seated toe grab

easy

① While seated, lean forward from your hips, relaxing your upper body on the inside of both thighs.

② Holding both feet with your hands, slowly exhale, pulling your chest down between your legs.

③ Relax from the stretch with your arms and inhale deeply as you return to a seated position again.

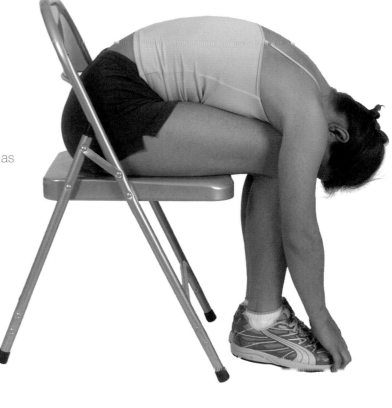

beach ball

easy

① Keeping your back straight, extend your arms in front of you at shoulder height, slightly bent.

② Place one hand in front of the other, palms facing you.

③ Slowly exhale, pushing your inner hand out while pulling your outer hand inward, making a circle with your arms.

④ Lower your head during the stretch. Inhale and relax your arms before raising your head.

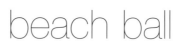

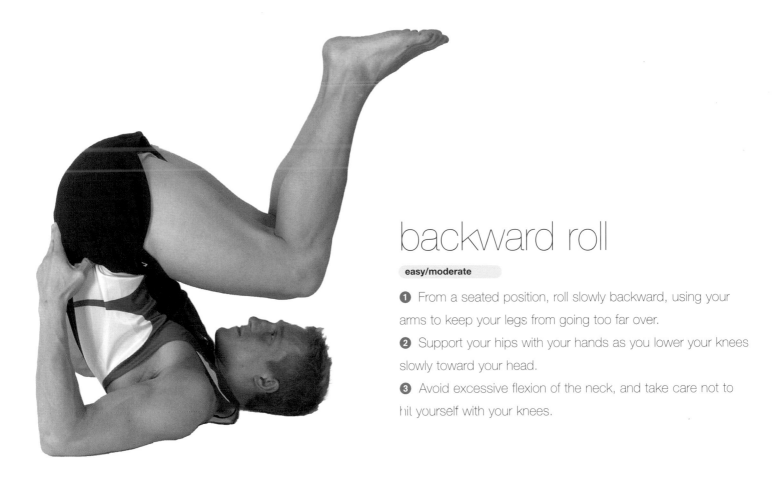

backward roll

easy/moderate

❶ From a seated position, roll slowly backward, using your arms to keep your legs from going too far over.

❷ Support your hips with your hands as you lower your knees slowly toward your head.

❸ Avoid excessive flexion of the neck, and take care not to hit yourself with your knees.

upper back **extended prayer**

easy/moderate

❶ From a kneeling position, extend both hands out, fingers pointing forward.

❷ Use your hands and forearms to grip the floor, as you gently ease your buttocks backward until you feel the stretch in your upper back and shoulders.

❸ Exhale, gently easing your chest down toward the floor.

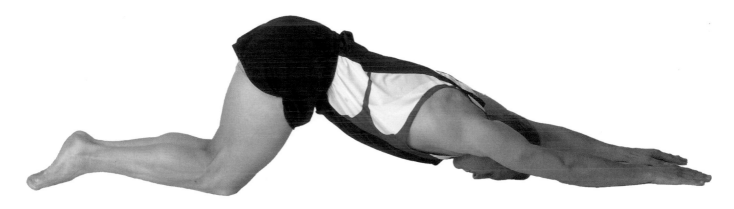

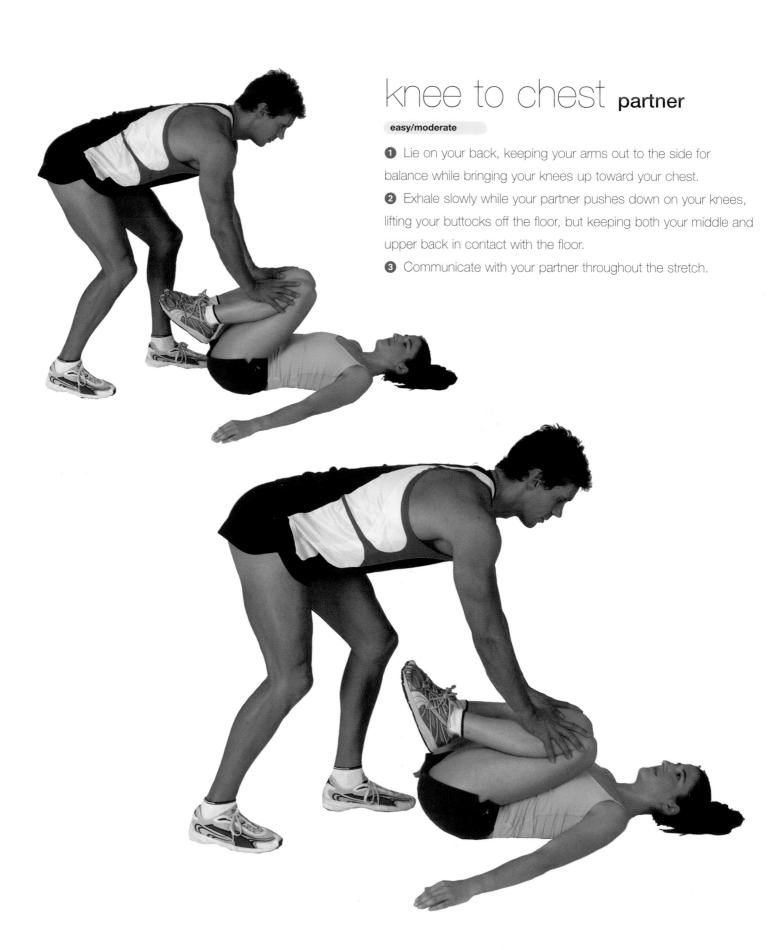

knee to chest **partner**

easy/moderate

1 Lie on your back, keeping your arms out to the side for balance while bringing your knees up toward your chest.

2 Exhale slowly while your partner pushes down on your knees, lifting your buttocks off the floor, but keeping both your middle and upper back in contact with the floor.

3 Communicate with your partner throughout the stretch.

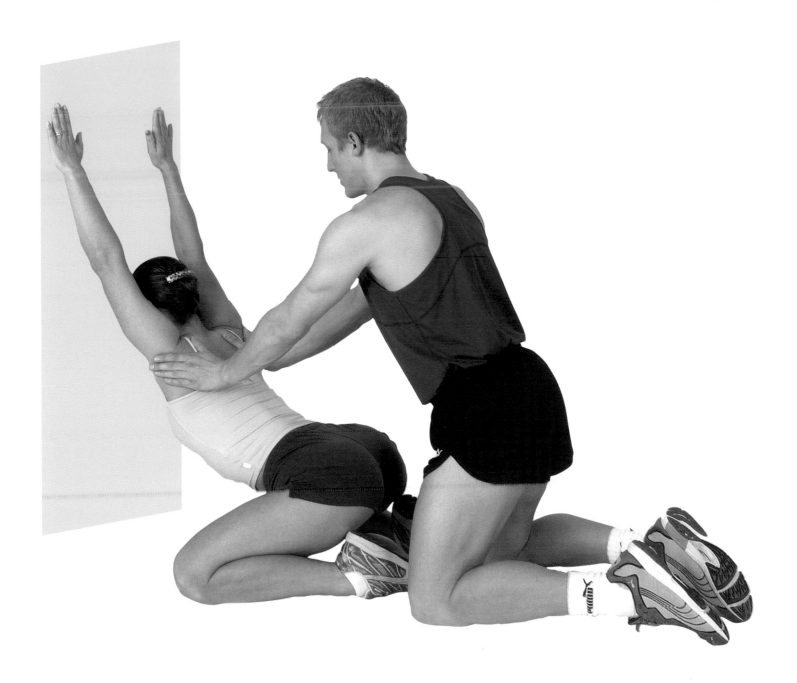

upper back **partner push**

moderate

❶ Place both palms on a wall, arms straight in a kneeling position, with your knees spread wide, sitting on your feet.

❷ Communicate with your partner while he pushes down on your shoulder blades as you exhale.

❸ You can adjust the hand position so that your palms are to the side to also feel the stretch in your chest and shoulder muscles.

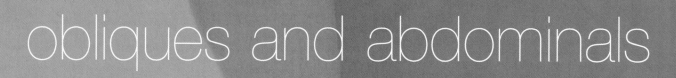

obliques and abdominals

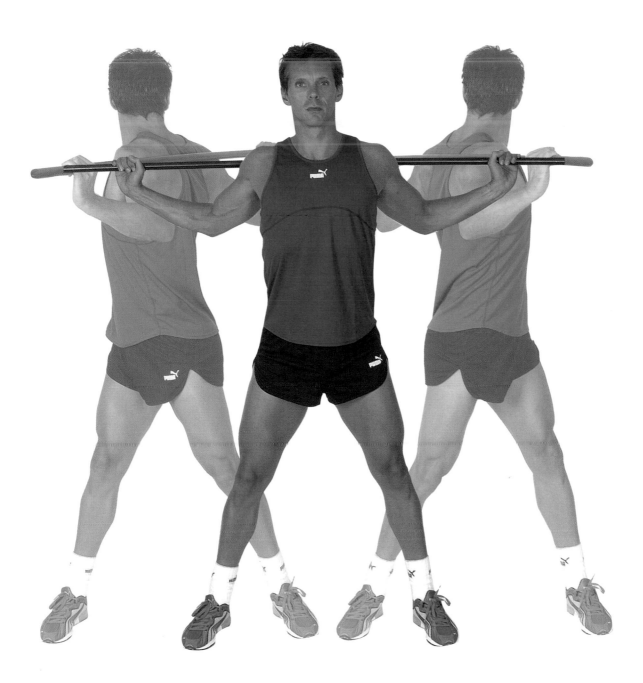

bar twist

easy

1 Stand with both feet facing forward, a double shoulder width apart, with legs slightly bent.

2 Use the bar to keep your upper body straight with elbows high, as you slowly twist around in both directions.

3 Avoid moving too quickly or forcing the stretch.

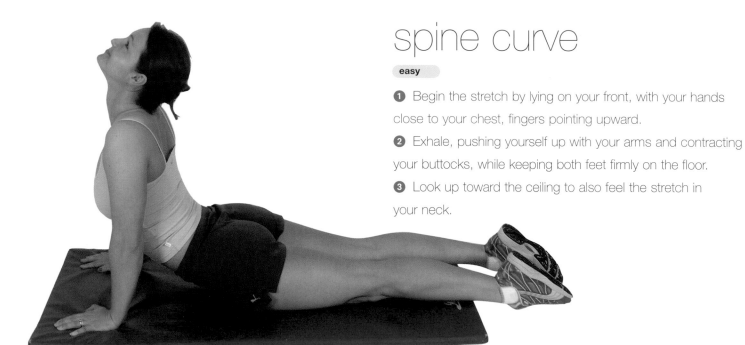

spine curve

easy

❶ Begin the stretch by lying on your front, with your hands close to your chest, fingers pointing upward.

❷ Exhale, pushing yourself up with your arms and contracting your buttocks, while keeping both feet firmly on the floor.

❸ Look up toward the ceiling to also feel the stretch in your neck.

trunk twist **seated**

easy

❶ Sit comfortably on a chair, raising both elbows high, hands clasped together.

❷ Inhale, slowly twisting to one side, keeping your back straight throughout the movement.

❸ Breathe comfortably while feeling the stretch.

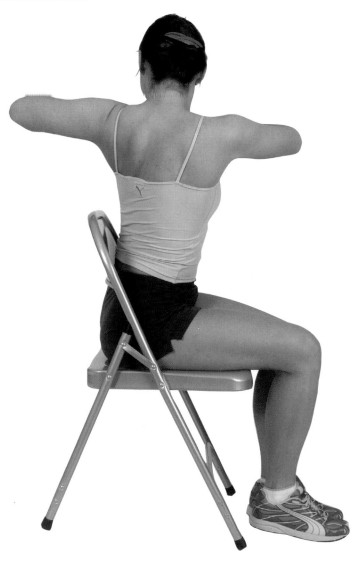

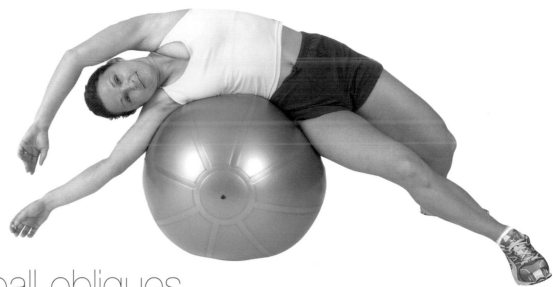

exercise ball obliques

easy/moderate

❶ Rest the side of your body, from your hip to your underarm, along the top of a suitable exercise ball.

❷ Keep your lower leg straight and slightly forward, and your other leg bent, with the foot behind to aid balance.

❸ Exhale, lowering your top arm over your head, down toward the floor.

❹ Stay relaxed on the ball, allowing the weight of your arms to control the stretch.

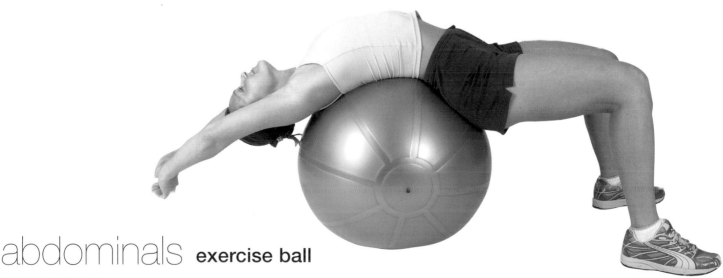

abdominals **exercise ball**

easy/moderate

❶ Rest on an exercise ball that allows your buttocks and shoulder blades to keep in contact with the ball.

❷ Your feet should be shoulder width apart, with the soles in contact with the floor.

❸ Exhale, taking both arms over your head, allowing gravity to pull your arms slowly toward the ground.

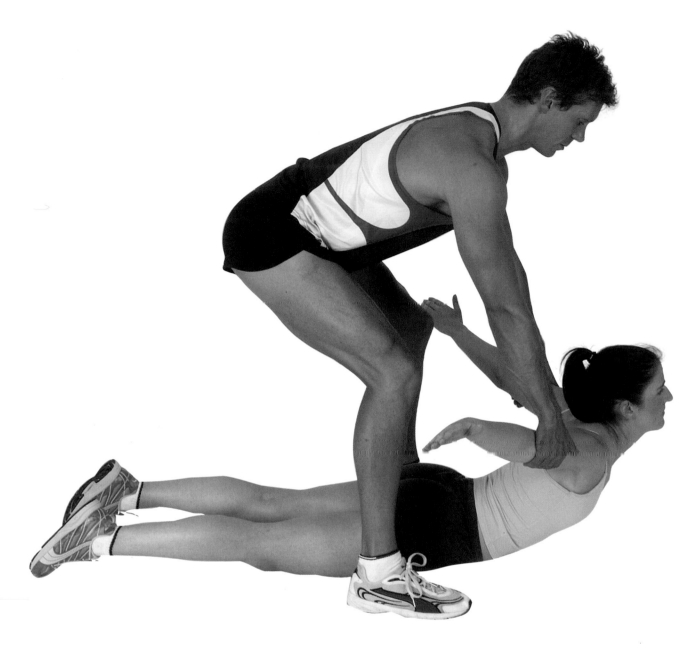

partner high dive

easy/moderate

❶ Lie on your chest with both arms extended straight out to the sides.

❷ Your partner will be standing outside of your hips, grasping both arms between your biceps muscle and elbow joint.

❸ As you slowly inhale, your partner will gradually lift your chest off the floor, aiming for an arch in your spine.

❹ Contract your buttocks and keep your feet on the floor throughout the lift.

❺ There needs to be good communication between partners, making sure that both the lift and the lower are performed under control.

back arch

moderate/hard

1 Bring both heels up toward your hips while resting your hands by your ears, fingers pointing down toward your toes.

2 Inhale and lift your body upward. Martial artists may wish to rest their head on the floor to stretch the neck muscles as well.

3 Make sure the surface is nonslip and that you lift your neck prior to relaxing the position.

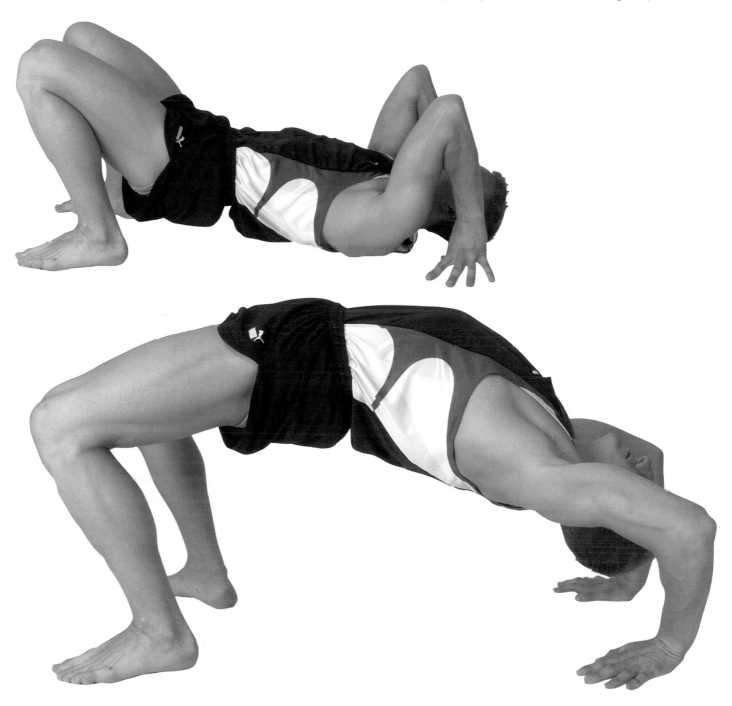

bar hang

easy/moderate

1 Hang from a secure bar with both hands, keeping your feet in contact with the floor, ideally one pace back from the bar.

2 Exhale, gently pushing your pelvis forward, keeping your arms and legs straight.

lying trunk twists

easy/moderate

1 Lie flat on your back with both hands extended straight out to your sides.

2 Slide both legs up toward one arm, keeping the knees together, while allowing your lower body to naturally twist around.

3 Can be performed with either bent or straight legs.

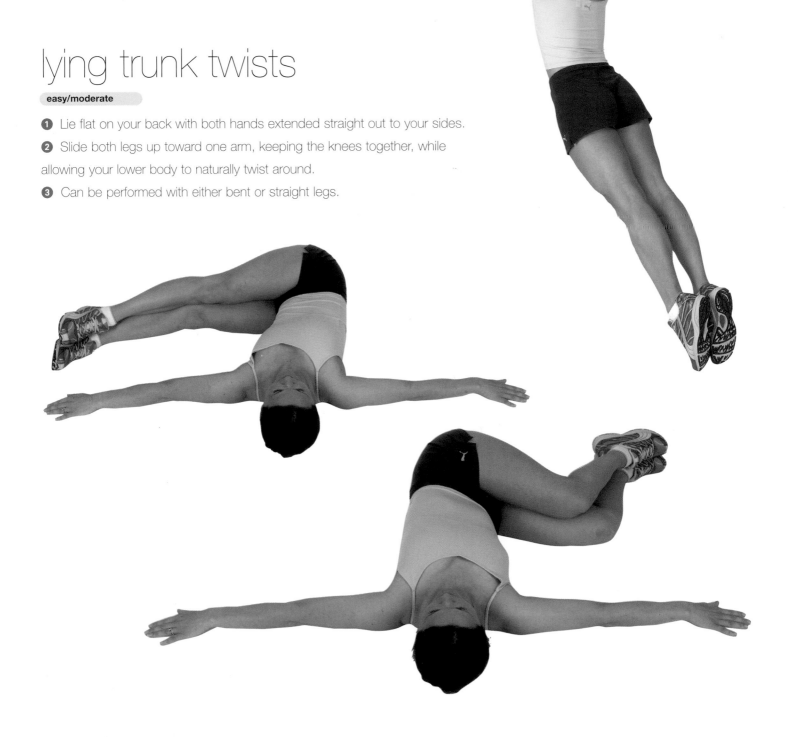

parachute

moderate

❶ Lie face down on the floor, taking both hands behind your back to grab either your foot or ankle.

❷ Inhale while slowly lifting your chest and knees off the floor, keeping your buttocks tensed and head looking upward slightly.

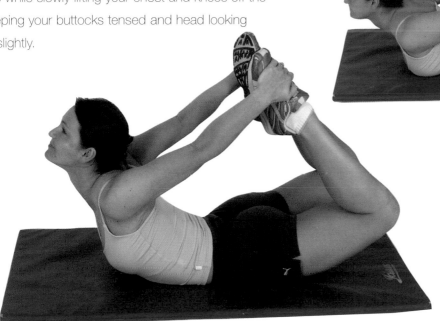

looking at ceiling

moderate

❶ Begin the stretch by kneeling on the floor, holding your heels with both hands.

❷ Slowly exhale, lifting your buttocks up and forward while taking the head backward in order to arch the back.

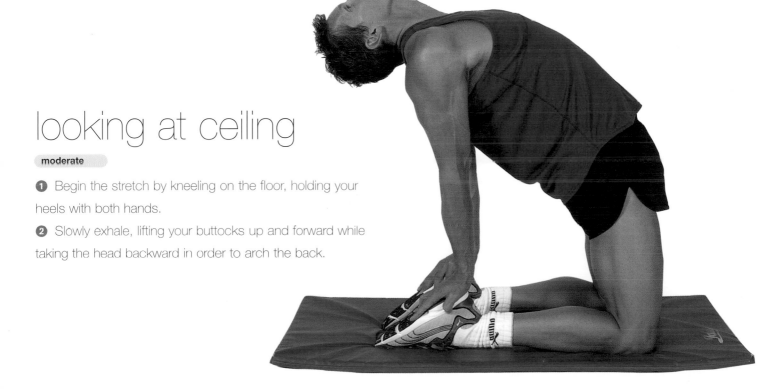

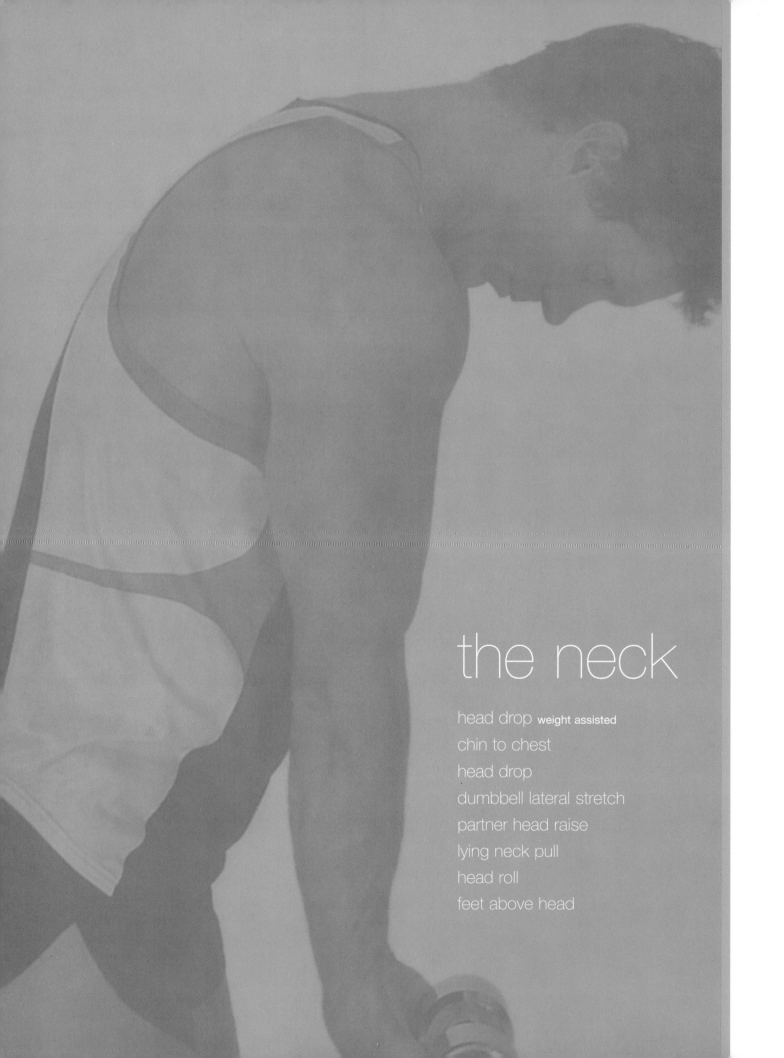

the neck

head drop **weight assisted**

chin to chest

head drop

dumbbell lateral stretch

partner head raise

lying neck pull

head roll

feet above head

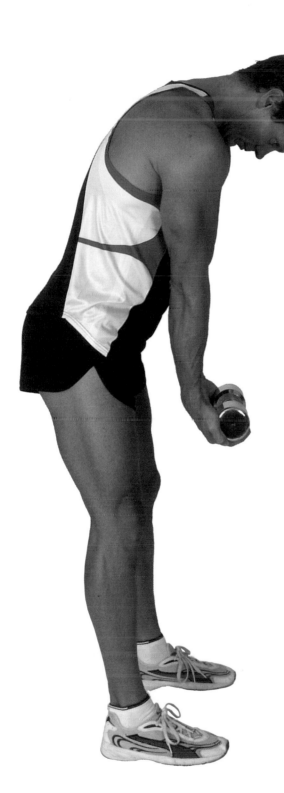

head drop weight assisted

easy

❶ Stand or sit on the edge of a chair, holding a light weight in both hands, either to the front or side of your hips, keeping your arms straight.

❷ Slowly exhale, lowering your chin to your chest and your shoulders to the floor.

❸ Avoid leaning forward excessively and keep your back straight throughout.

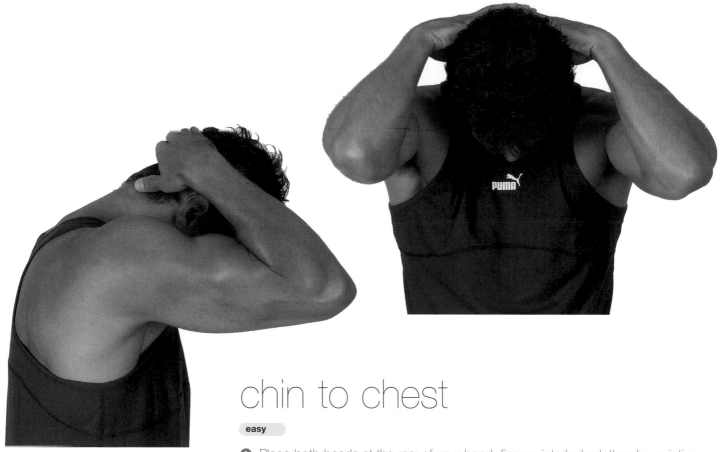

chin to chest

easy

❶ Place both hands at the rear of your head, fingers interlocked, thumbs pointing down, elbows pointing straight ahead.

❷ Slowly exhale, pulling your head downward, aiming for your chin to touch your chest.

❸ Concentrate on keeping your back straight with your shoulders down and back.

❹ Relax your hands and inhale as you lift your head.

head drop

easy/moderate

❶ Rest on a raised platform on your back with your head and neck extended over the edge.

❷ Exhale, lowering your head down slowly toward the floor, keeping your shoulders in contact with the platform.

❸ Inhale, slowly lifting your head upward after your stretch.

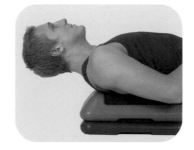
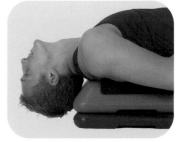

dumbbell lateral stretch

easy

❶ Stand, holding a light weight in one hand.

❷ Exhale slowly, allowing your head to drop down toward the shoulder of the weighted arm and feeling the stretch on the free hand side of your neck.

❸ Progress this stretch by using your free hand to slowly pull your head down toward the shoulder of your free hand, feeling the stretch on the weighted side.

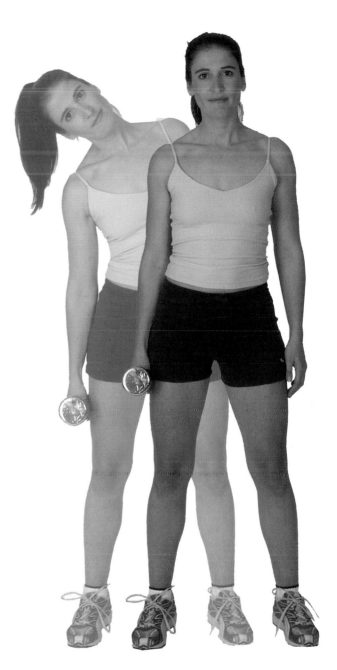

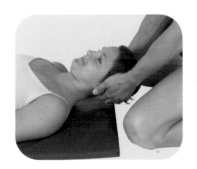
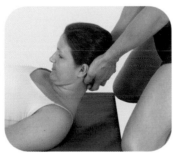

partner head raise

easy/moderate

❶ Lie on the floor while your partner lightly holds your head on either side of your ears.

❷ Communicate with your partner as you slowly exhale while he gently lifts your head, taking your chin to your chest.

❸ Relax back down, controlling the movement and keeping your shoulders in contact with the floor at all times.

❹ This stretch can also be performed on a raised platform with your head hanging over the edge in order to stretch the front of your neck.

lying neck pull

easy/moderate

❶ Lie on your back with both legs bent, feet firmly on the floor.

❷ Grasp the back of your head with your fingers, resting your palms on the top of your head.

❸ Exhale, slowly pulling your chin down toward your chest, keeping your upper back in contact with the floor.

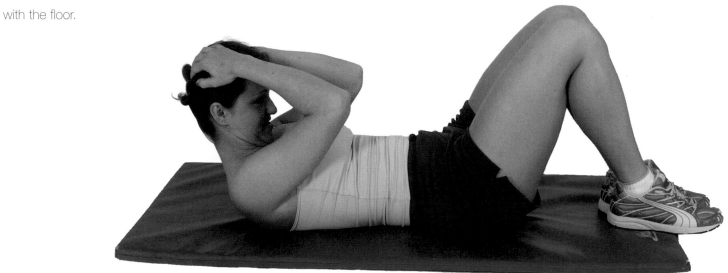

head roll

moderate/hard

❶ Kneel on all fours, placing your forearms on the floor with your head resting on its crown between your elbows.

❷ Slowly and gently roll your shoulders forward as your chin comes closer to your chest.

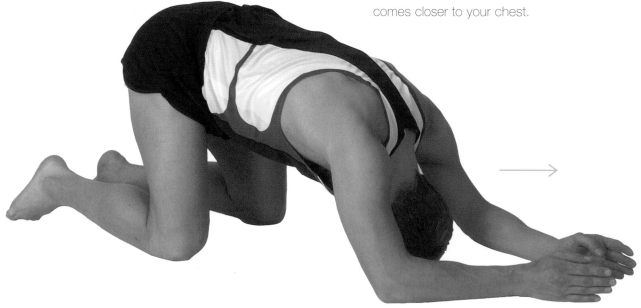

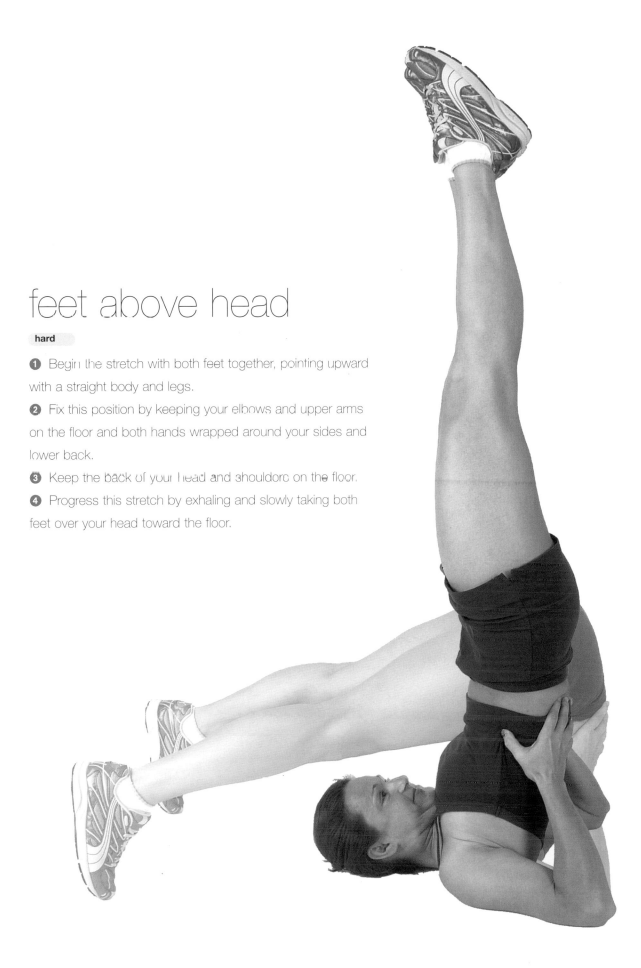

feet above head

hard

1 Begin the stretch with both feet together, pointing upward with a straight body and legs.

2 Fix this position by keeping your elbows and upper arms on the floor and both hands wrapped around your sides and lower back.

3 Keep the back of your head and shoulders on the floor.

4 Progress this stretch by exhaling and slowly taking both feet over your head toward the floor.

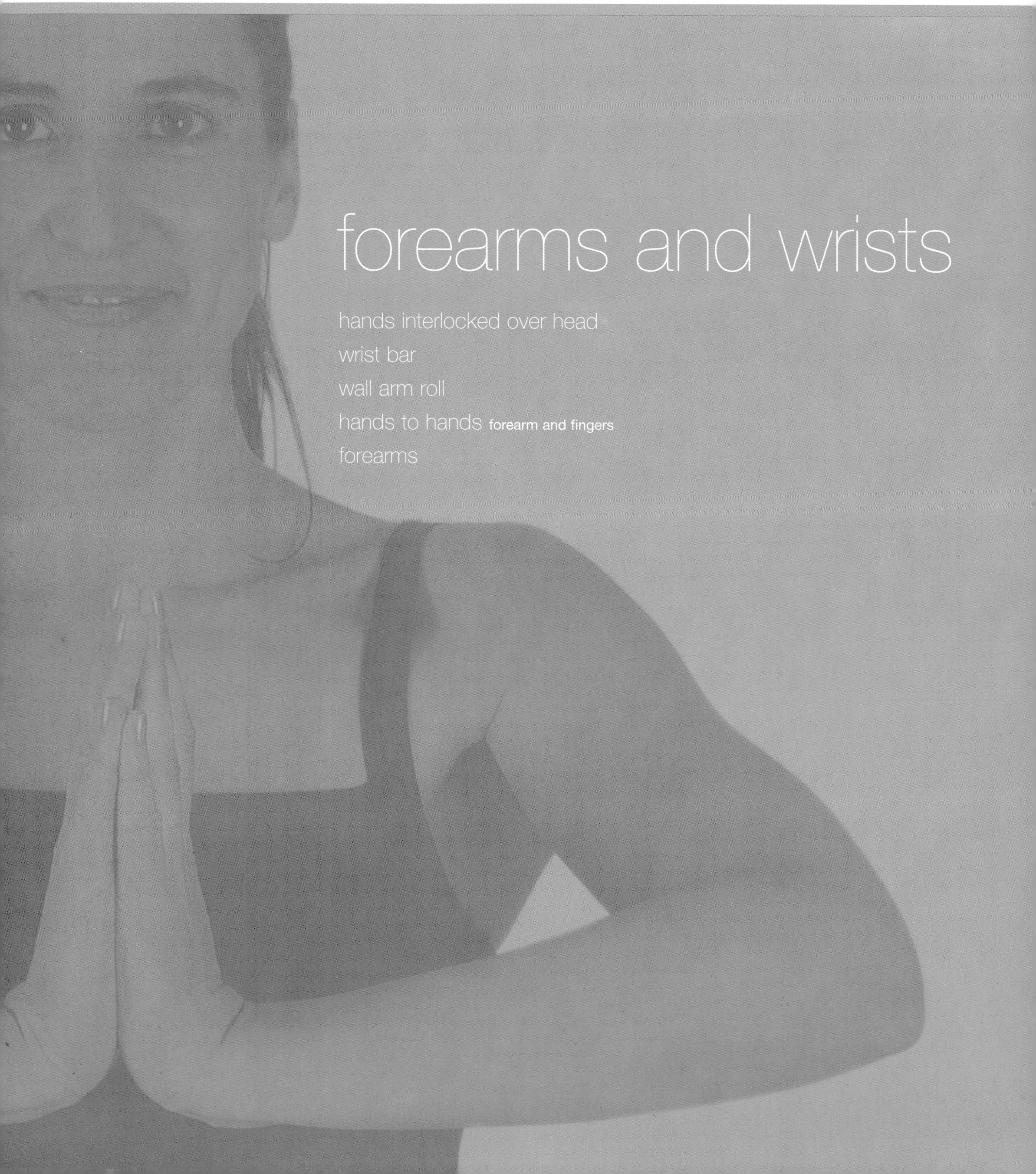

forearms and wrists

hands interlocked over head

wrist bar

wall arm roll

hands to hands **forearm and fingers**

forearms

hands interlocked over head

easy

① Interlock your fingers above your head, palms facing upward.

② Exhale and push your hands further above your head.

③ You will also feel this stretch in your shoulders.

wrist bar

easy/moderate

① Hold a bar or broomstick with your palms facing upward, fingers wrapped around the bar, thumbs pointing away from the body.

② Exhale, slowly lifting the bar by bending the arms while keeping the wrists in contact with the bar.

③ Can be performed with a narrow, normal, or wide grip.

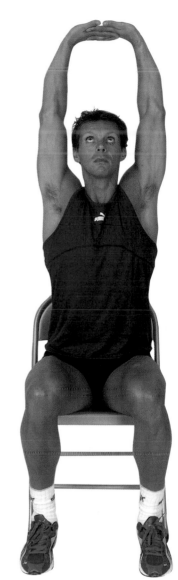

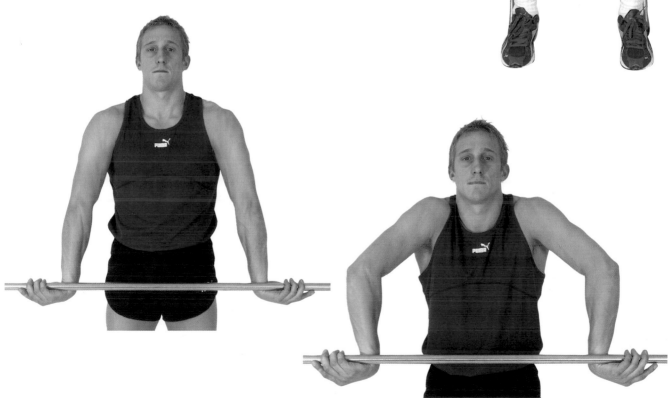

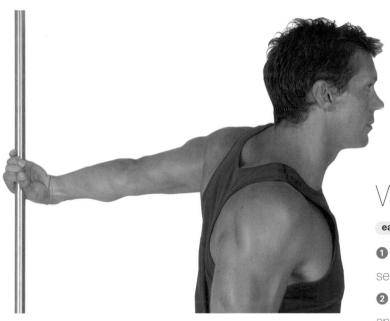

wall arm roll

easy

1 Extend one arm behind, grasping onto a pole or similar secure object.

2 Your arm should be straight with your elbow facing upward, and your thumb underneath your fingers.

3 Exhale, slowly rolling your arm around so that your elbow faces the floor.

hands to hands **forearm and fingers**

easy

1 Place both palms and fingers together, keeping your elbows high.

2 Exhale and push hands hard together. Your fingers should slowly part with only your palms and fingertips touching.

3 While in the same position, you can lower your fingers to one palm and gently push your hands together to stretch your fingers.

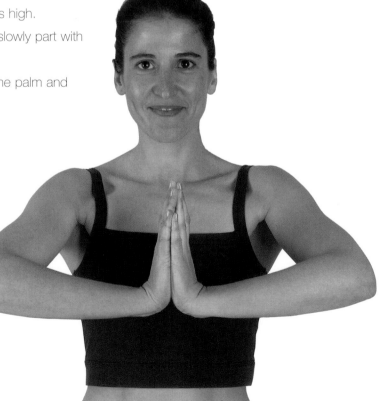

forearms

easy

❶ Kneel on all fours, using a combination of hand positions to stretch the many different muscles in the wrists and forearms.

❷ Gently ease into the stretch by pushing your shoulders either back or forward.

❸ Variations of this stretch are to point the fingers outward, inward, or forward.

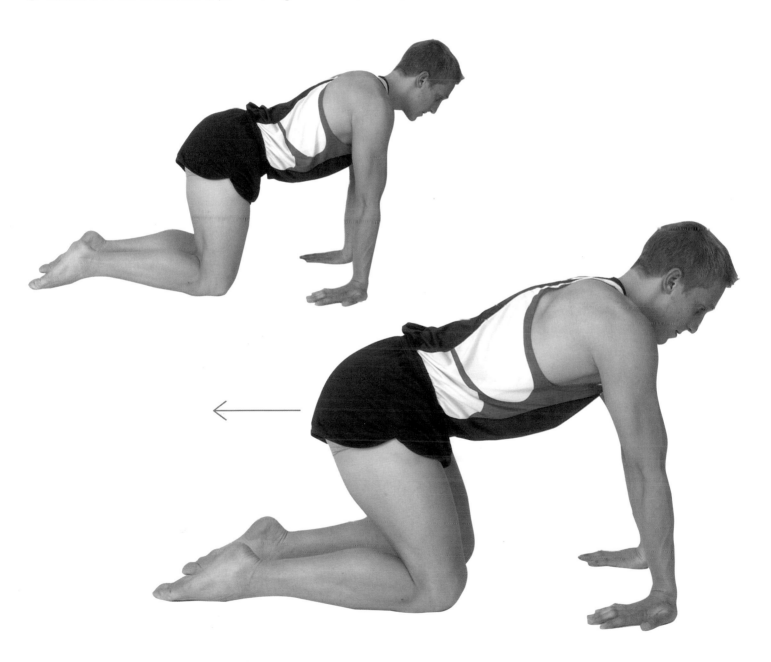

triceps and biceps

triceps **partner**

❶ While seated, extend one arm down the center of your spine, elbow pointing upward.

❷ Your partner will pull down gently on your wrist while pushing down gently on your elbow.

❸ Exhale slowly, communicating with your partner throughout the stretch.

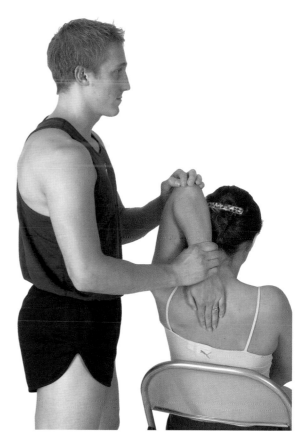

triceps dip

❶ Place your hands on the edge of a secure chair with your fingers pointing forward.

❷ With your legs extended out to the front, lower your buttocks to the floor.

❸ Hold the position when your arms are in the downward phase in order to feel the stretch.

❹ Avoid holding too long, as you will not be able to rise again.

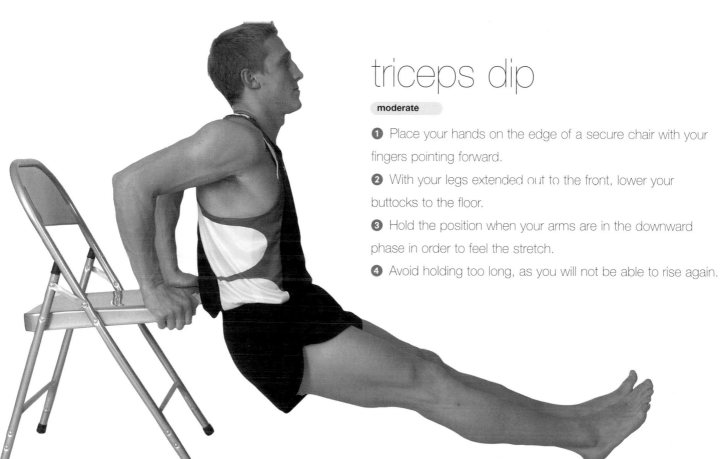

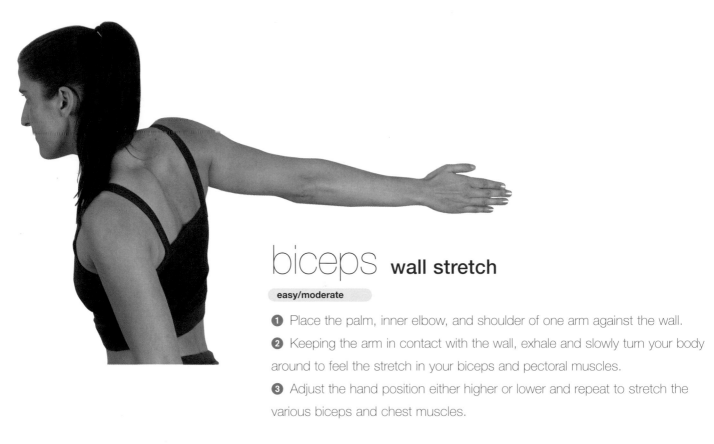

biceps **wall stretch**

easy/moderate

❶ Place the palm, inner elbow, and shoulder of one arm against the wall.

❷ Keeping the arm in contact with the wall, exhale and slowly turn your body around to feel the stretch in your biceps and pectoral muscles.

❸ Adjust the hand position either higher or lower and repeat to stretch the various biceps and chest muscles.

biceps **weight assisted**

easy

❶ Sit on a chair with one hand crossed on the opposite leg, placing your palm on the thigh.

❷ Holding a light weight in the other hand, keep the arm straight between your legs, resting on your forearm against your wrists.

❸ Allow the weight to straighten your arm while keeping your back straight and shoulders back.

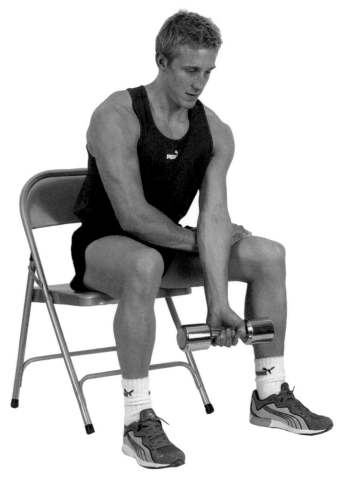

triceps

easy/moderate

❶ Extend one hand down the center of your back, fingers pointing downward.

❷ Use the other hand to grasp the elbow.

❸ Exhale slowly, pulling gently downward on your elbow, taking your fingers along your spine.

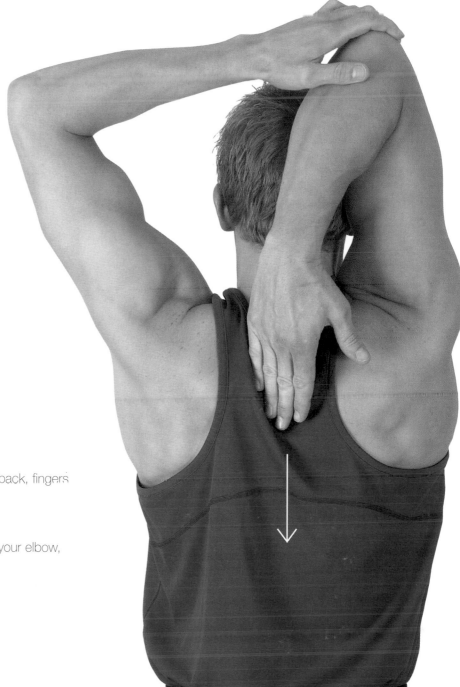

triceps interlock

moderate/hard

1 Extend one arm down your back, fingers bent, palm facing your spine.

2 Bend your other arm behind your back, palm facing outward with your fingers bent.

3 Grasp both hands with your fingers.

4 Exhale, pulling on both arms, keeping the fingers interlocked.

5 Be careful if you have long fingernails.

6 If you can't grasp your hands, use a towel.

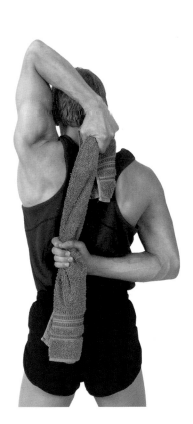

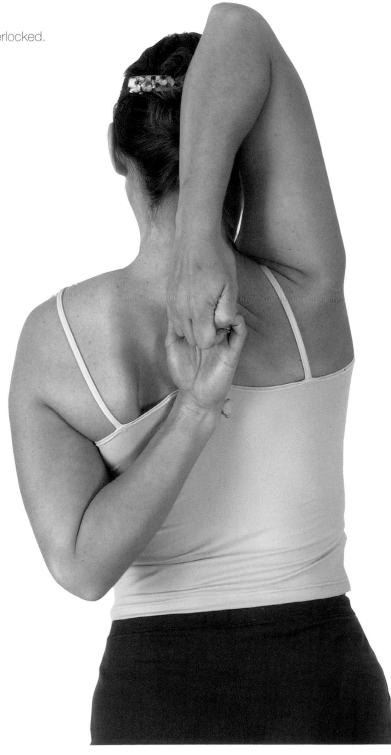

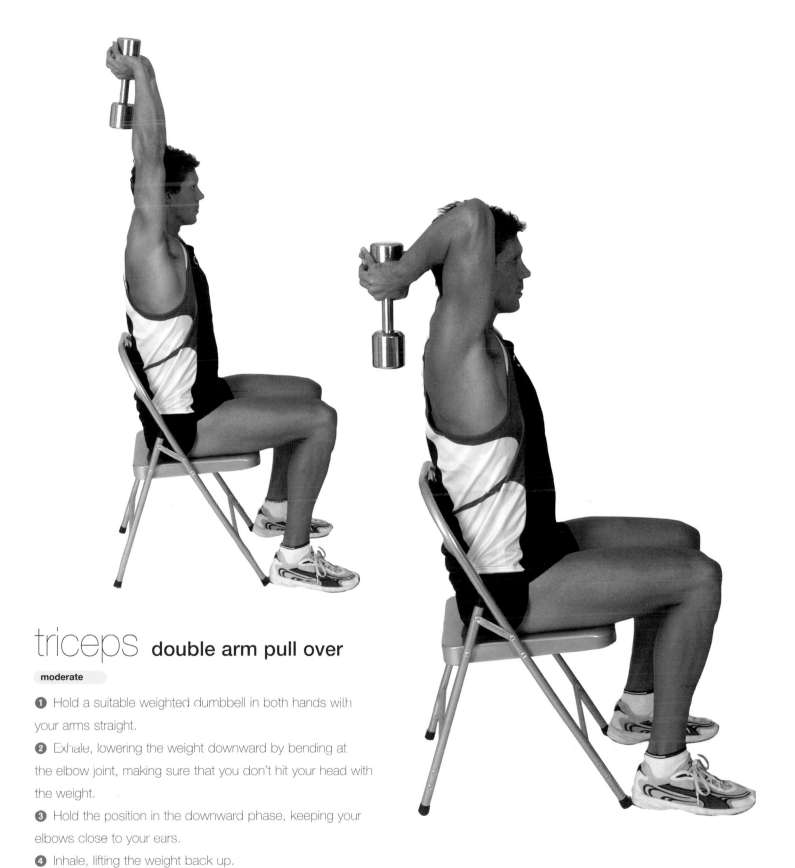

triceps **double arm pull over**

moderate

❶ Hold a suitable weighted dumbbell in both hands with your arms straight.

❷ Exhale, lowering the weight downward by bending at the elbow joint, making sure that you don't hit your head with the weight.

❸ Hold the position in the downward phase, keeping your elbows close to your ears.

❹ Inhale, lifting the weight back up.

❺ Avoid using a weight that is too heavy, and, if necessary, have a partner take the weight from you in the downward phase.

shoulders

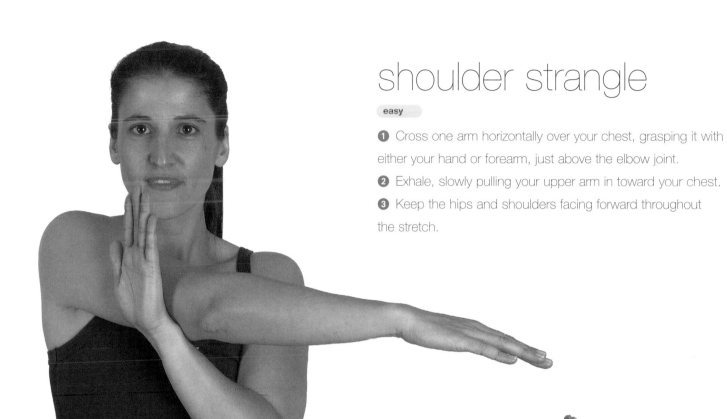

shoulder strangle

easy

❶ Cross one arm horizontally over your chest, grasping it with either your hand or forearm, just above the elbow joint.

❷ Exhale, slowly pulling your upper arm in toward your chest.

❸ Keep the hips and shoulders facing forward throughout the stretch.

hand lock with forearms

moderate

❶ Cross both arms straight out in front of you.

❷ Bend the lower arm up and over the upper arm, aiming to grasp the upper palm with the fingers of your lower arm.

❸ Exhale, slowly turning your forearms and wrists, so that your thumbs are facing you.

❹ Increase the stretch by lowering both elbows.

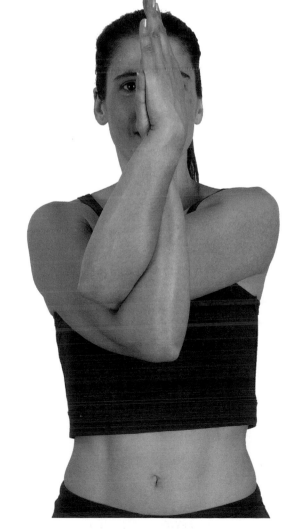

backward prayer

moderate

❶ Stand or sit with both arms behind your back, placing the tips of your thumbs and fingers together, pointing upward.

❷ Inhale, slowly pushing your palms together.

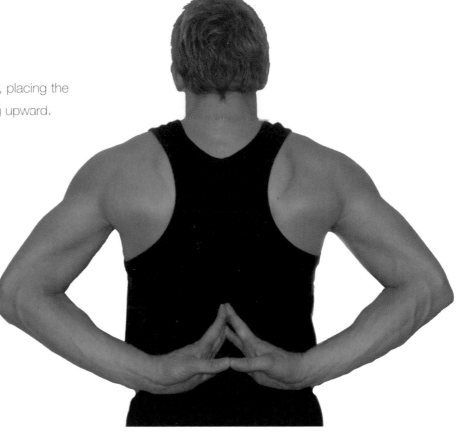

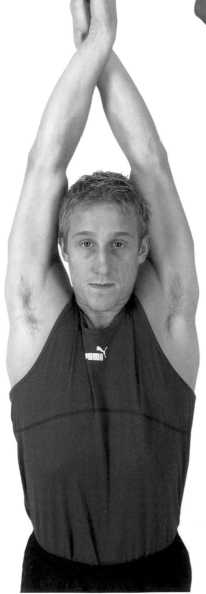

upward stretch

easy

❶ Extend both hands straight above your head, palms touching.

❷ Inhale, slowly pushing your hands upward, then backward, keeping your back straight.

❸ Exhale and relax from the stretch before you repeat.

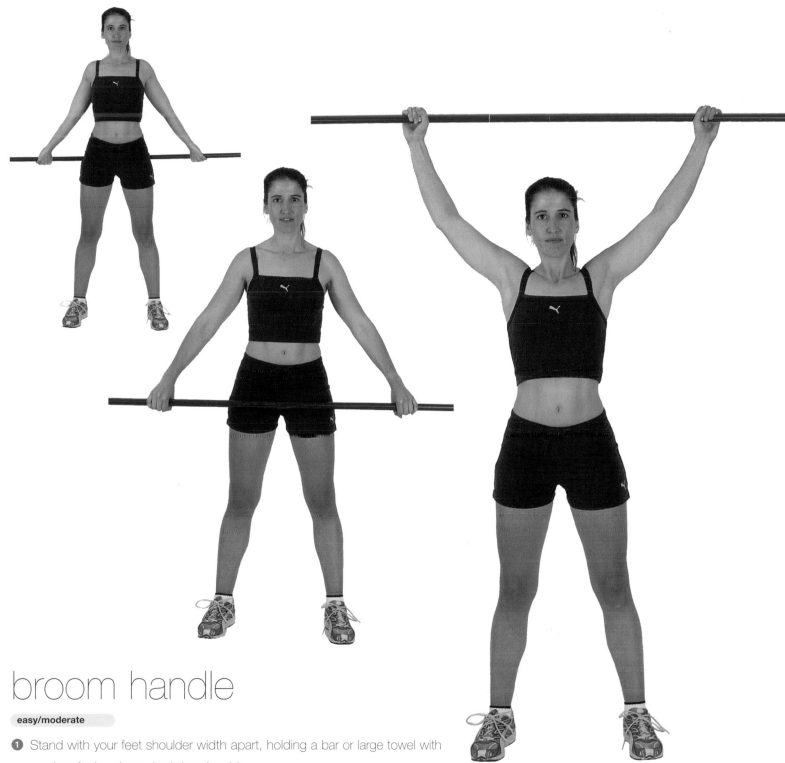

broom handle

easy/moderate

❶ Stand with your feet shoulder width apart, holding a bar or large towel with your palms facing down, both hands wide.

❷ Inhale, slowly take both arms behind your head, resting your hands at either side of your hips, palms facing behind.

❸ You may find that one arm needs to bend as you twist to the side in order to perform this stretch. Concentrate on avoiding this; simply work within your limits.

arm arrest

easy/moderate

1 Extend both arms behind your back, grasping one of your elbows.

2 Exhale, slowly pulling the grasped elbow toward your spine.

3 Hold your wrist if you are unable to reach your elbow.

4 Dropping your head down toward your shoulder will also stretch your neck.

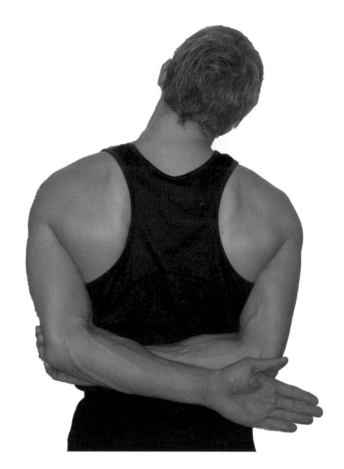

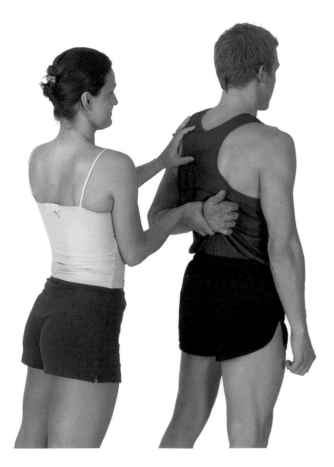

shoulder arm arrest **partner**

moderate

1 Stand with one arm behind your back, palm facing outward.

2 Your partner will grasp your wrist with one hand, while the other is pressed against the shoulder blade of the bent arm.

3 Communicate with your partner as he slowly pulls your bent arm upward, taking your hand toward the opposite shoulder.

reverse prayer

moderate

❶ Sit or stand with both hands behind your back, palms together and fingers pointing upward.

❷ Your partner will hold both your arms on the outside of the elbow.

❸ Communicate with your partner as he slowly pulls back on your elbows, keeping your palms and fingers together.

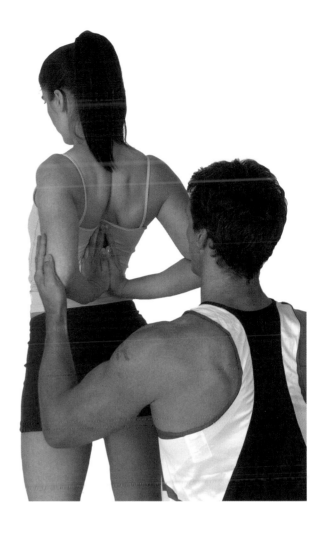

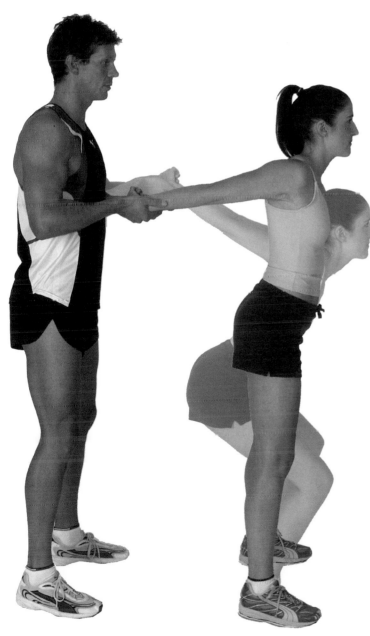

partner shoulder pull

easy/moderate

❶ Stand with both your hands grasped behind you by your partner, keeping your arms straight.

❷ Communicate with your partner, as you slowly lower yourself by bending your legs while your partner applies upward pressure on your arms.

❸ Relax from the stretch by standing upright, and then repeat, going further down in order to develop the stretch.

shoulders **exercise ball**

moderate

❶ Lie on an exercise ball or bench with arms straight above your head, holding a light weight to increase the stretch.

❷ Inhale, slowly lowering your arms to either side of your head, keeping your arms straight.

❸ Hold the stretch in the downward phase, breathing comfortably throughout, gradually lowering the weight toward the floor.

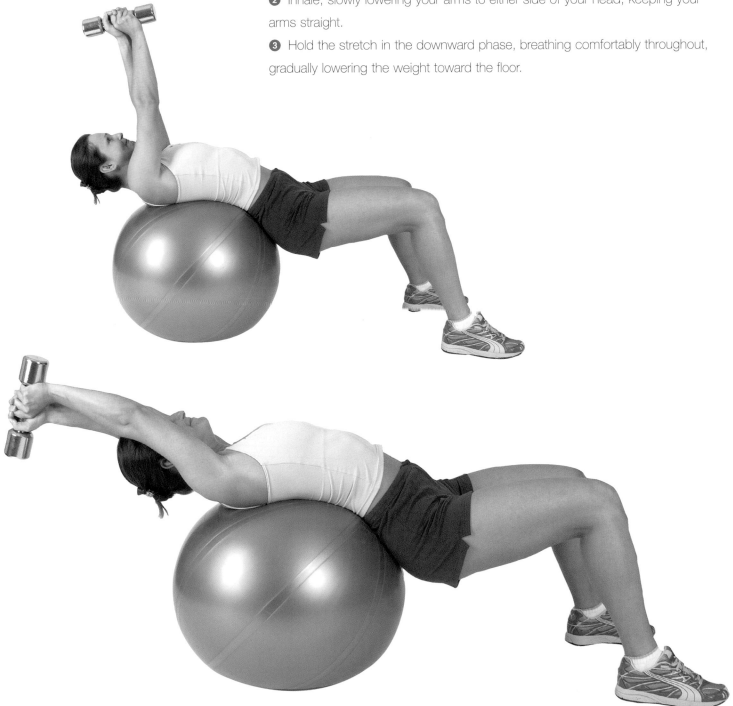

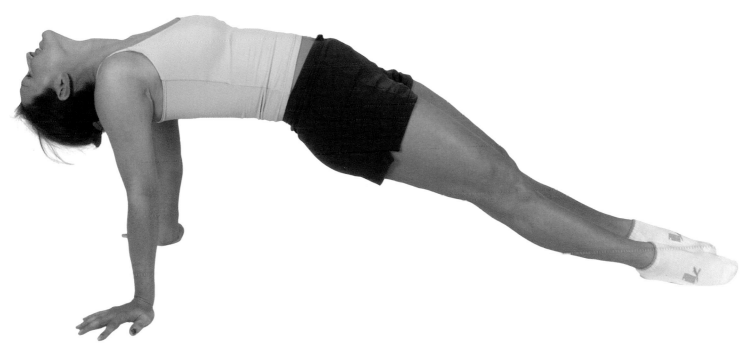

reverse push-up

moderate/hard

❶ Sit on the floor with your feet extended straight out in front of you.

❷ Your hands should be behind you, palms flat on the floor, fingers pointing out to the sides, in line with your shoulders during the upward phase.

❸ Inhale, lifting your buttocks off the floor, taking your head back, resting only on your hands and heels.

❹ Raise your head prior to lowering yourself back down, making sure you control the movement.

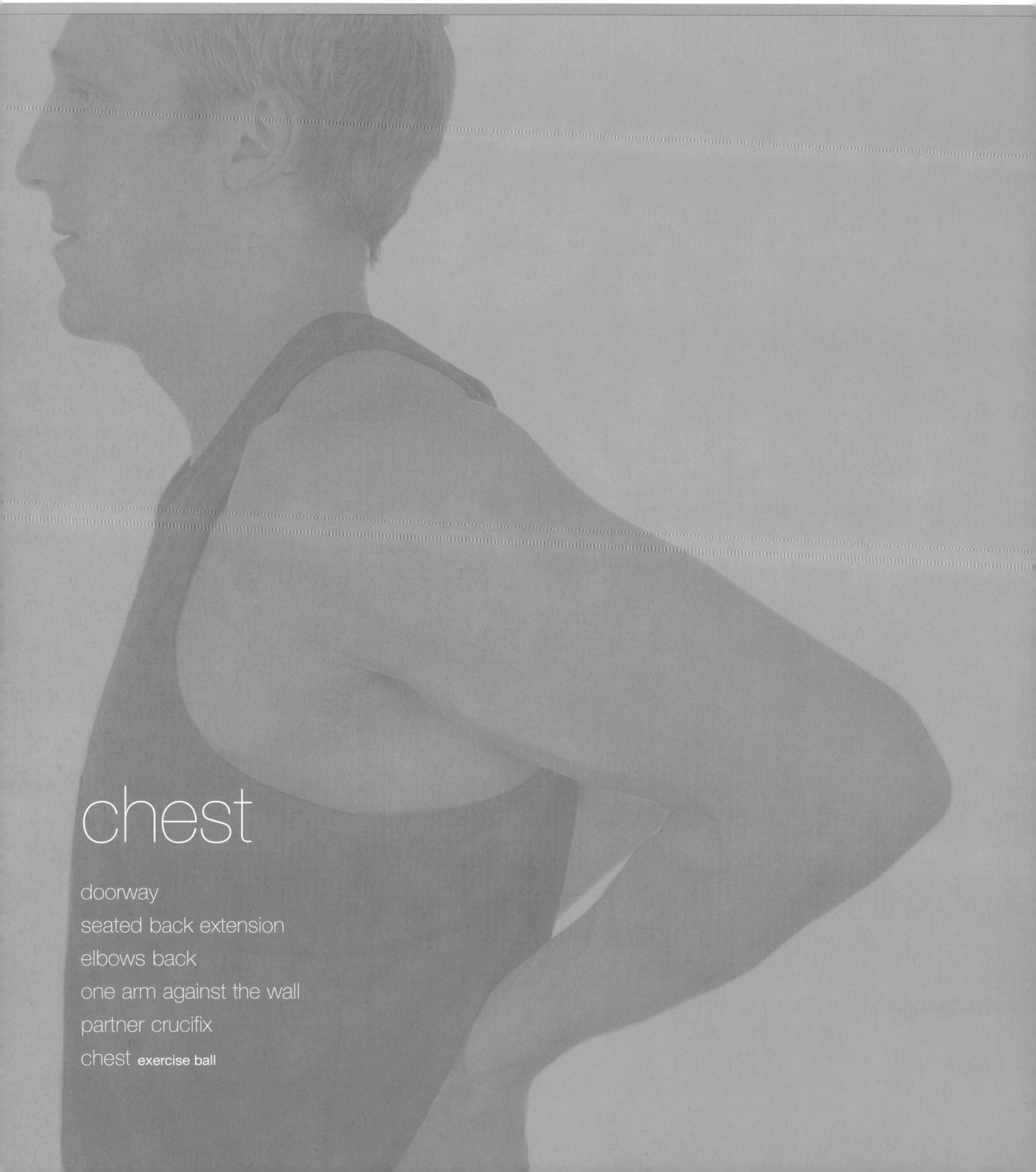

chest

doorway

seated back extension

elbows back

one arm against the wall

partner crucifix

chest **exercise ball**

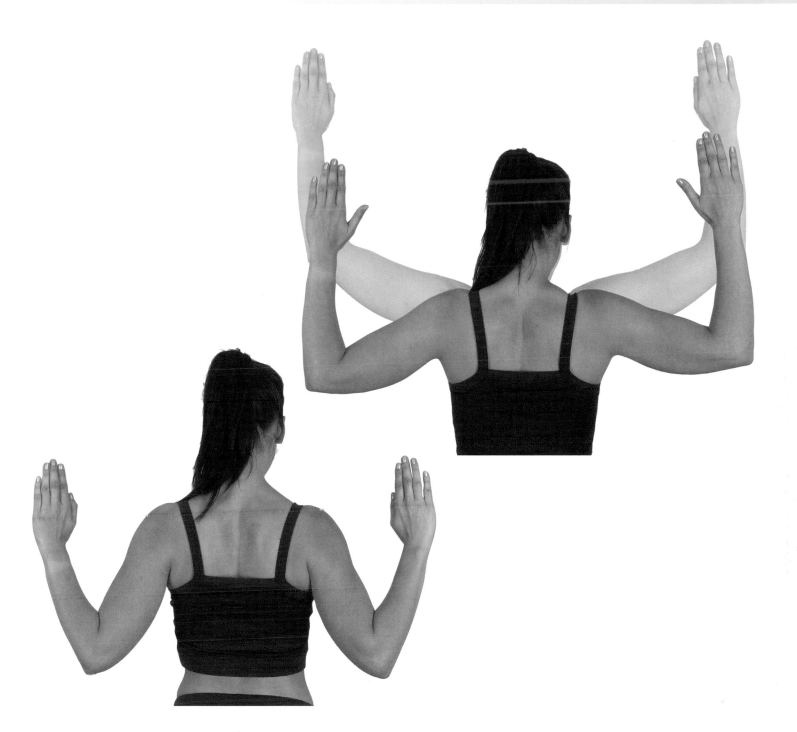

doorway

easy

❶ Stand in a doorway, placing your forearms and palms in contact with the door frame.

❷ Exhale, slowly pushing your chest through the doorway, keeping your arms firmly on the frame.

❸ You can adjust the position of your hands to work different muscle fibers of the chest (pectoral) muscles.

seated back extension

easy

❶ Sit on a chair, feet firmly on the floor under your knees.

❷ Lock your hands behind your head, keeping your elbows high and extended back.

❸ Inhale, pushing your chest forward and upward while arching the spine and taking your elbows further back.

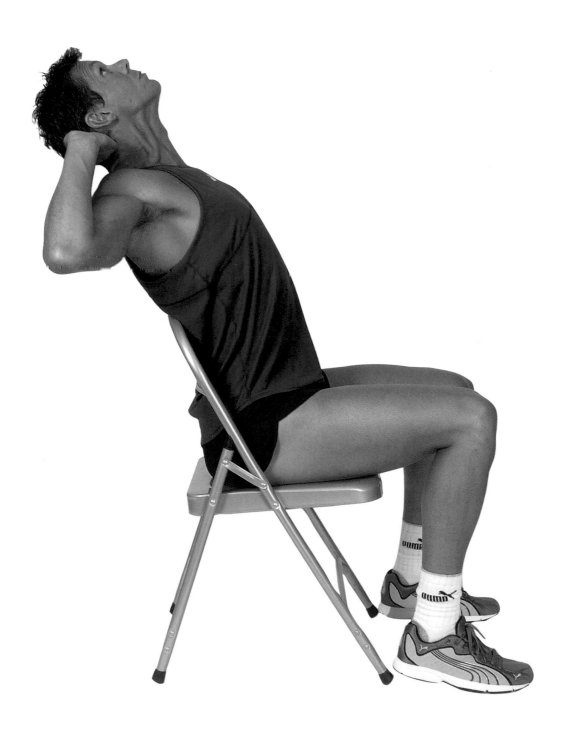

elbows back

easy

❶ Stand or sit upright, keeping your back straight, head looking forward.

❷ Place both hands on your lower back, fingers pointing downward, elbows out to your side.

❸ Exhale slowly while gently pulling the elbows back, aiming to get them to touch.

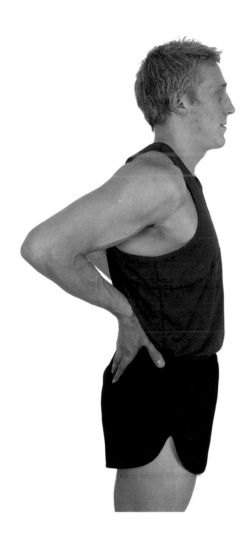

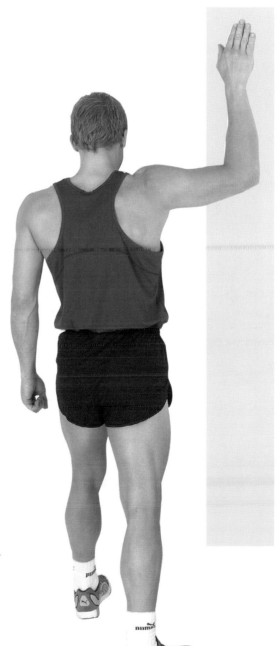

one arm against the wall

easy/moderate

❶ Place your forearm and biceps against a wall, keeping the arm at right angles.

❷ Exhale, slowly turning your opposite shoulder backward, keeping the other arm firmly in contact with the wall.

❸ Repeat this stretch both raising and lowering the walled arm in order to work the different pectoral muscles.

partner crucifix

moderate

1 Sit with your arms either extended out to your sides or with your hands grasped behind your head.

2 Communicate with your partner as he pulls your arms back at the elbow joint.

3 Remember to exhale as you apply the stretch.

4 You can also perform this stretch with one arm, using the other arm to fix yourself into the chair, to avoid twisting.

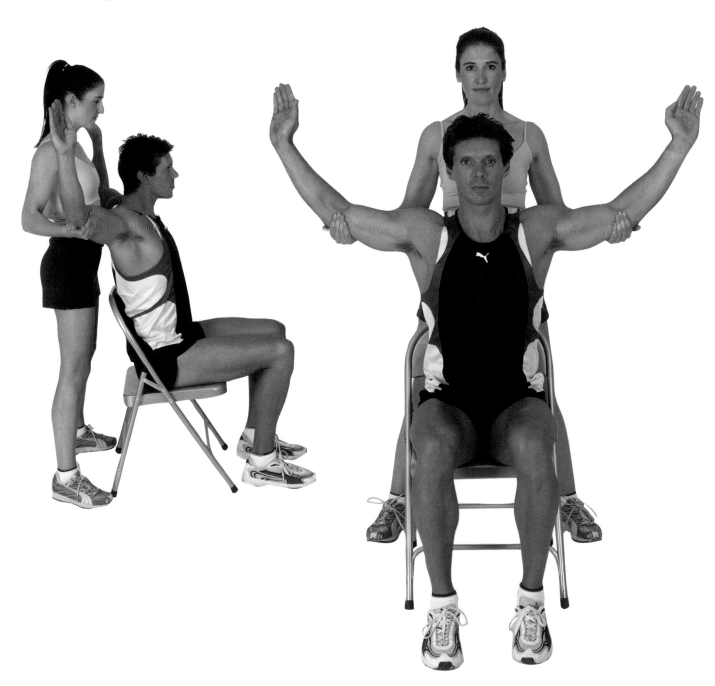

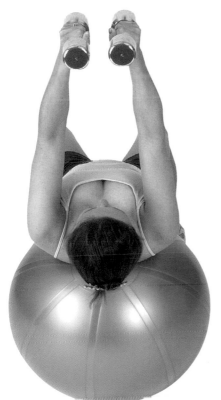

chest **exercise ball**

moderate/hard

1 Relax on either a bench or large exercise ball, placing your feet wide and firmly on the ground to give you good balance.

2 Holding a light dumbbell in each hand, slowly lower the weights from above your chest, out to your sides at shoulder level.

3 Breathe comfortably while in the downward phase, holding the weights in this position to feel the stretch.

4 Keep a slight bend in the elbows.

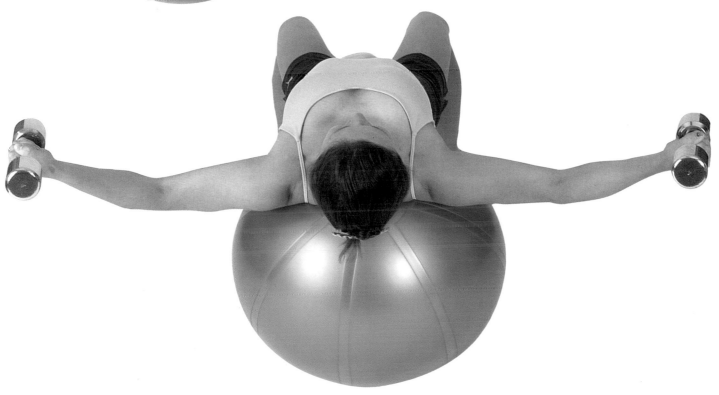

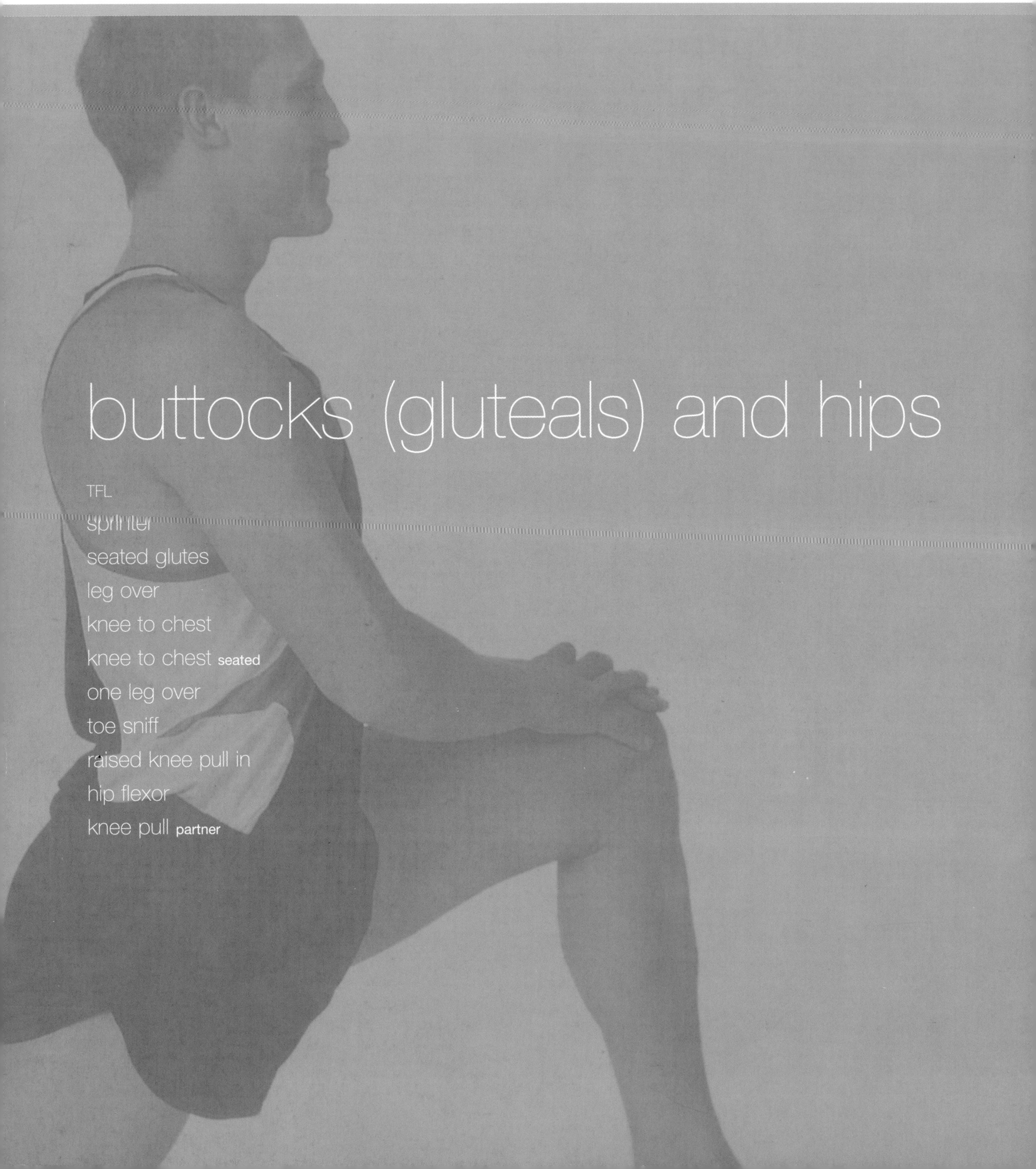

buttocks (gluteals) and hips

TFL

sprinter

seated glutes

leg over

knee to chest

knee to chest **seated**

one leg over

toe sniff

raised knee pull in

hip flexor

knee pull **partner**

TFL

easy

❶ Stand straight, placing one foot behind the other.

❷ Exhale, slowly lowering yourself a few inches down toward the back foot.

❸ Increase the stretch gradually by pushing the hip of the rear leg out to the side.

❹ Concentrate on keeping both legs straight with your feet in contact with the floor.

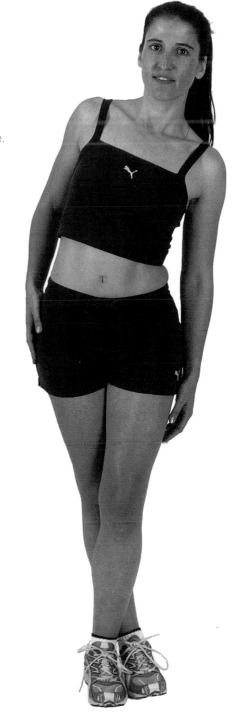

sprinter

hard

❶ Extend one leg straight back, resting the knee and front of the foot on the floor.

❷ Your front leg should be extended forward, keeping the sole of the foot in contact with the floor.

❸ Exhale, bending from your hips, aiming to place both your forearms on the floor while pushing your pelvis gently toward the floor.

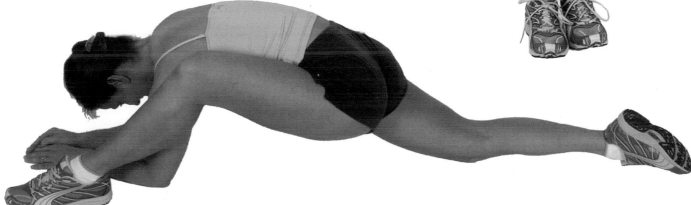

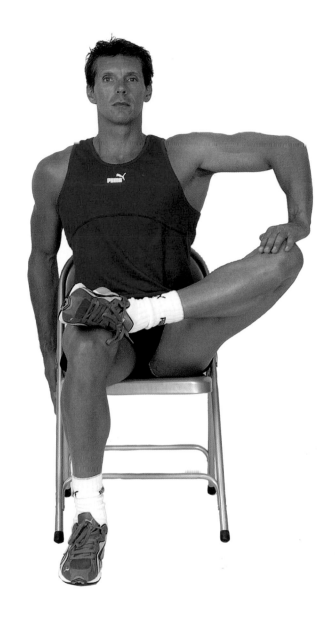

seated glutes

easy/moderate

❶ Sit with a straight back on a chair, with one leg crossed over and resting on your opposite thigh.

❷ Place one hand on the inside of the bent knee, and use the other to fix yourself into the chair.

❸ Exhale, slowly pushing down on the bent leg while gradually leaning forward.

leg over

moderate

❶ Lie on your back, extending your left arm out to the side while taking your left leg over your right and bringing the knee in line with your hips.

❷ Keeping your right leg straight, use your right arm to push down on the knee of the left leg, exhaling slowly as you stretch.

❸ Repeat for the other side.

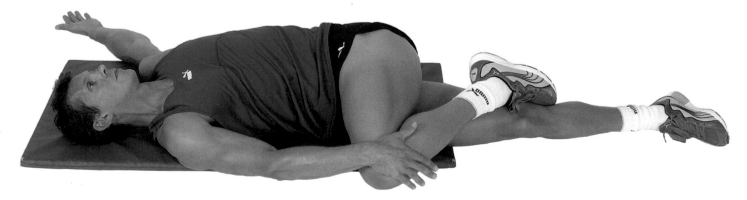

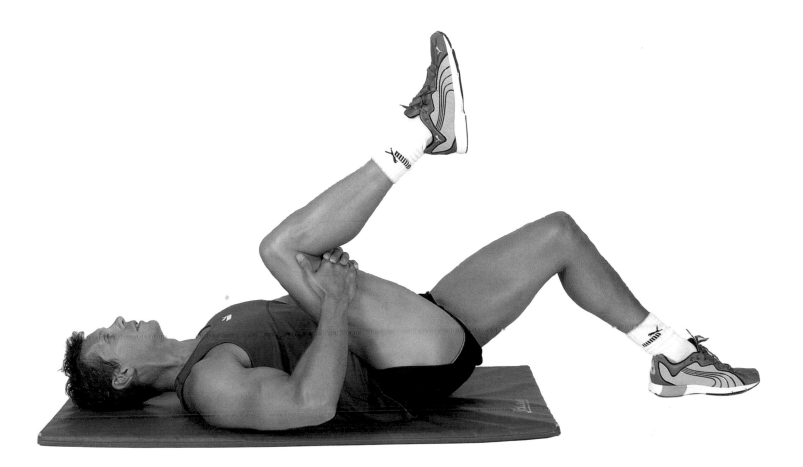

knee to chest

`easy`

1 Lie on your back and raise one leg, grasping it with both hands behind the knee.

2 Keep your head, shoulders, and other foot firmly on the floor.

3 Inhale, slowly pulling the raised leg toward your chest.

4 Repeat for the other side.

knee to chest **seated**

easy

❶ Raise one leg up onto a chair, resting your heel on the edge of the chair.

❷ Slowly pull the knee into your chest.

❸ Repeat the stretch again, this time taking the knee toward the chest and then across your body's centerline.

❹ Repeat using the other leg.

Work for one to three minutes.

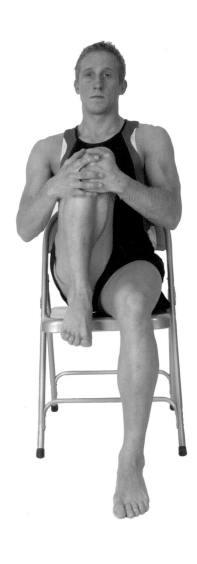

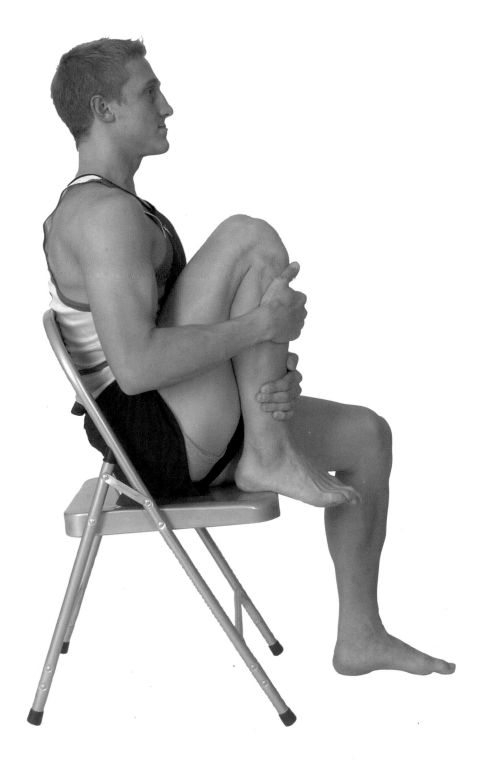

one leg over

moderate

1 Sit on the floor with one leg straight, toes pointing upward.

2 Cross the other foot over the knee of the straight leg, aiming to place that foot flat on the floor.

3 Place the elbow and forearm of the opposite arm of the bent leg on the outside of the bent knee.

4 Exhale, slowly pulling the bent knee across your body.

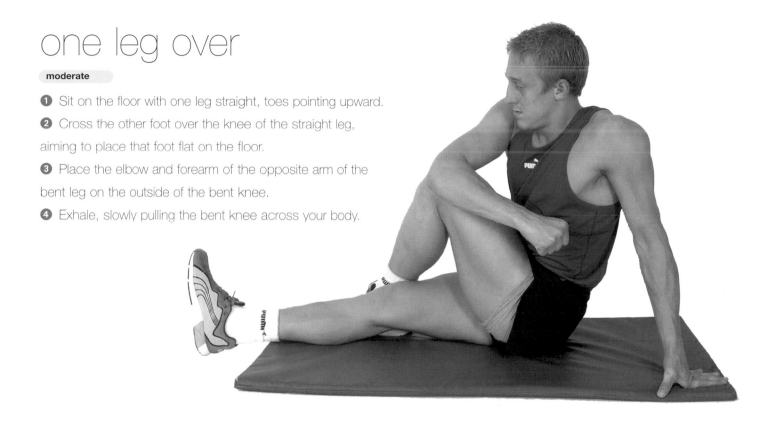

toe sniff

moderate/hard

1 Bend one leg, grasping the ankle and shinbone with both hands.

2 Keeping your back straight, exhale and pull the foot slowly up toward the opposite shoulder.

3 This stretch is best performed against a wall to aid your balance; alternatively, it can be done lying down.

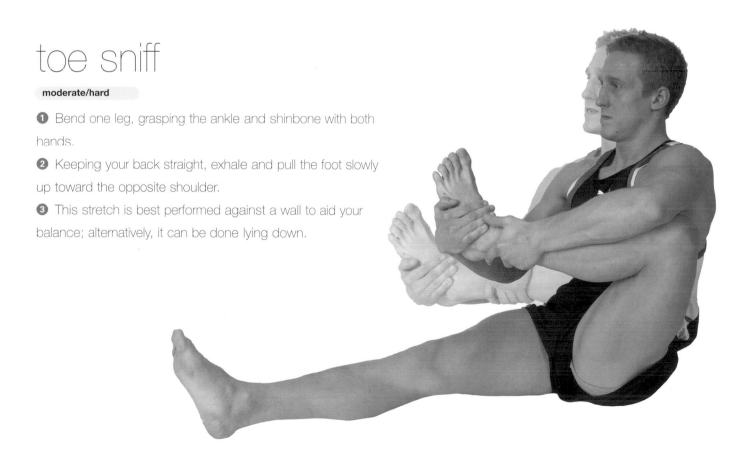

raised knee pull in

moderate

1 Lie on your back, lifting and bending one leg so it makes a right angle.

2 Place your other foot across the bent leg, using your hands if necessary. Aim to rest the foot above the knee on your thigh muscles.

3 Exhale, slowly pulling the bent leg toward you, keeping your upper back and head in contact with the floor.

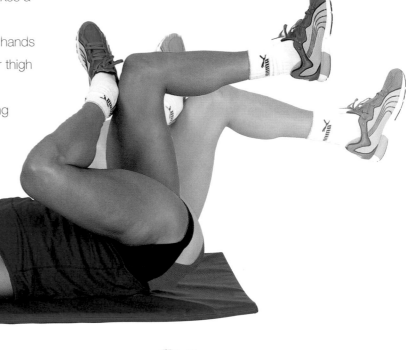

hip flexor

moderate

1 Rest one foot and knee on the floor, keeping your back straight.

2 Use your front leg for balance, as you push the thigh of the rear leg forward while tilting the pelvis upward.

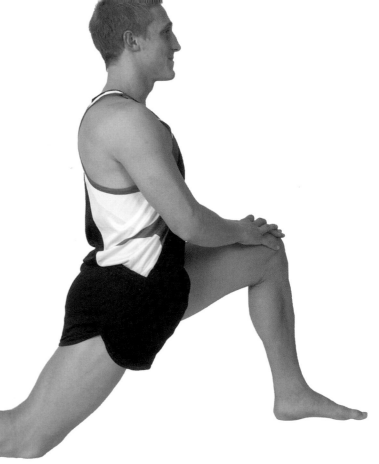

knee pull **partner**

moderate

❶ Lie flat down on your chest with one leg bent, foot facing upward.

❷ Your partner will grasp the bent leg under your knee, placing the other hand or forearm across the buttock of the bent leg.

❸ Communicate with your partner as he pushes down on your buttocks while pulling up at the knee.

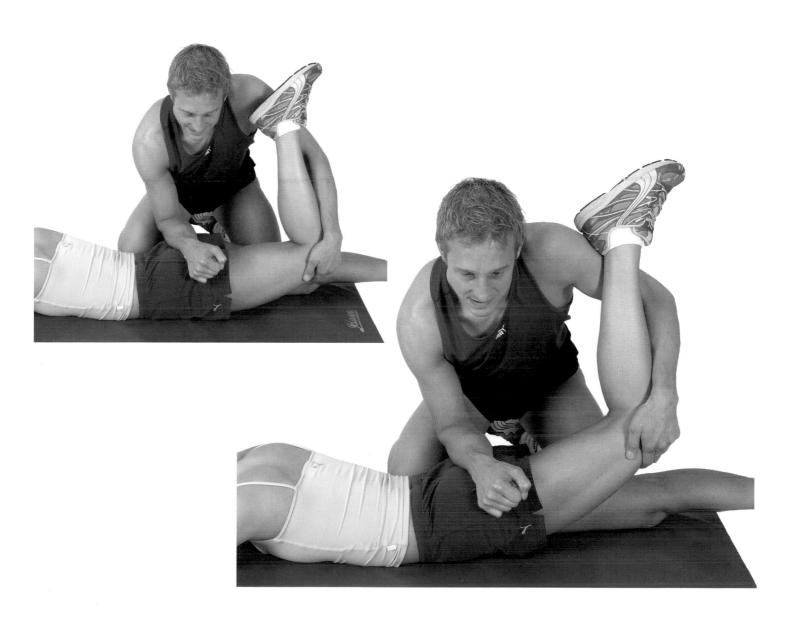

adductors

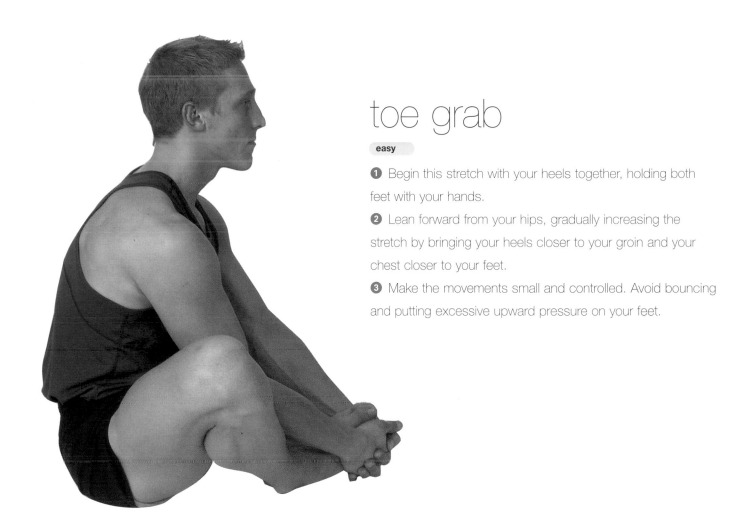

toe grab

easy

❶ Begin this stretch with your heels together, holding both feet with your hands.

❷ Lean forward from your hips, gradually increasing the stretch by bringing your heels closer to your groin and your chest closer to your feet.

❸ Make the movements small and controlled. Avoid bouncing and putting excessive upward pressure on your feet.

chair slump

easy

❶ Rest one foot on a secure raised platform, such as a chair, with the foot either facing forward or away from your body.

❷ The other foot should be one stride away from the raised foot, with the leg being straight.

❸ Exhale, slowly bending forward from your hips, and taking your hands down toward the floor.

❹ Avoiding bouncing, breathe comfortably while in the stretch position, returning up again using a slow, controlled movement.

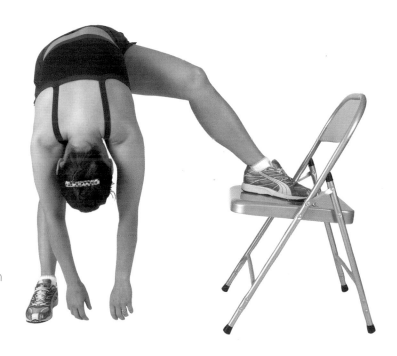

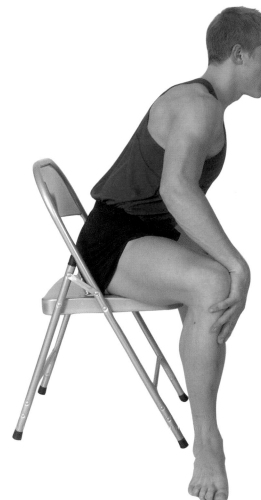

toes pointing at 180 degrees

moderate

❶ While seated, position your feet flat on the floor pointing the toes from each foot away from each other.

❷ Slowly extend your body forward from the hips while gradually pushing on the inside of your knees to increase the stretch.

frog position

easy/moderate

❶ With your heels shoulder width apart, feet facing outward, slowly squat down, placing your hands on the floor.

❷ Exhale, gradually push against the insides of your knees with your arms, and take the legs further apart while keeping both feet firmly on the floor.

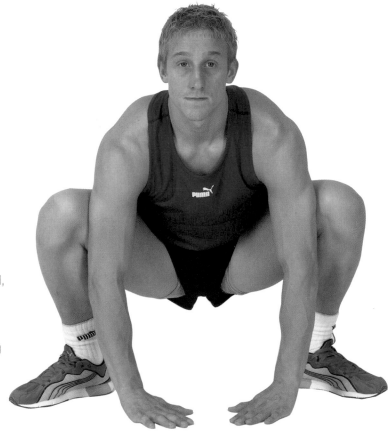

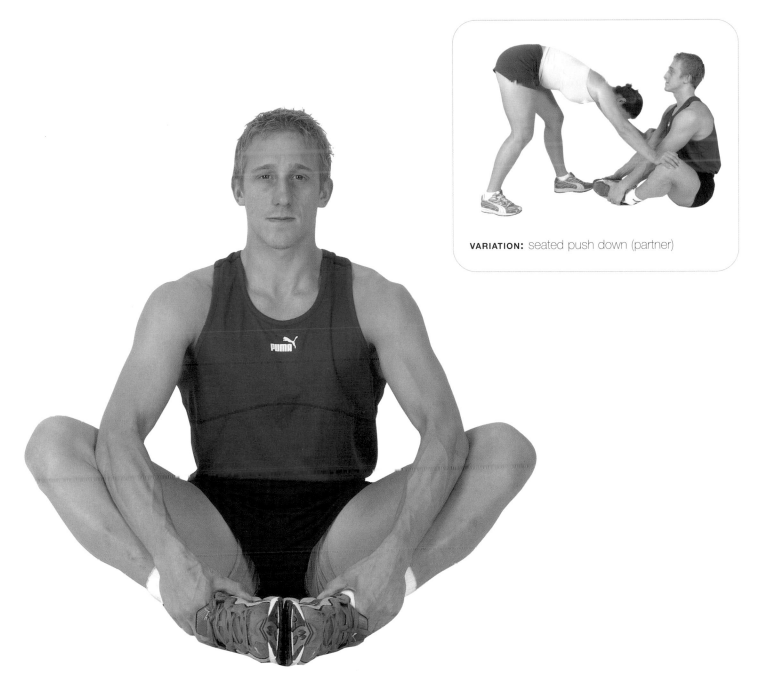

VARIATION: seated push down (partner)

elbows into knees

`easy`

❶ Sit on the floor, grab both feet around the ankles, and slowly pull them in toward your groin.

❷ Place your elbows against the inside of your knees, keeping your back straight throughout.

❸ Slowly exhale as you push downward with your elbows, gradually pushing the knees toward the floor.

❹ Relax the stretch for a few seconds and then repeat, taking the stretch slightly further.

❺ Sitting with your back pressed against a wall will help increase the stretch.

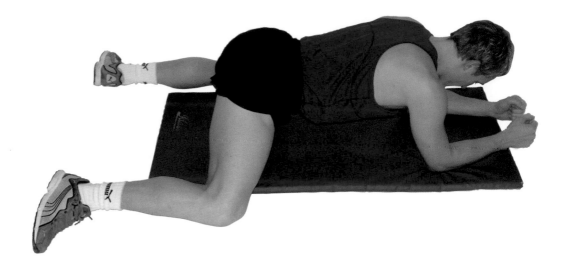

frog

moderate/hard

❶ Kneel on all fours, resting on your forearms with your knees spread wide, in line with your hips, with your feet behind your buttocks.

❷ Exhale, slowly lowering yourself to the floor, extending your arms forward while taking your feet out to the side, lowering your groin to the floor.

sitting legs straight partner

easy/moderate

❶ Sit on the floor with either of your hands behind you or your back against a wall.

❷ Your partner will be kneeling between your legs, which should be spread, feet pointing upward and legs straight.

❸ Slowly exhale as your partner pushes your legs apart with their hands on your lower leg.

❹ Communicate with your partner throughout the stretch.

side lunge

easy

❶ Stand upright, with both feet facing forward, double shoulder width apart.

❷ Place your hands on your hips in order to keep your back straight and slowly exhale, taking your body weight across to one side.

❸ Avoid leaning forward or taking the knee of the bent leg over your toes. As you increase the stretch, the foot of the bent leg should point slightly outward.

❹ To increase the stretch, relax upward, slowly sliding the straight leg out a few inches and repeating.

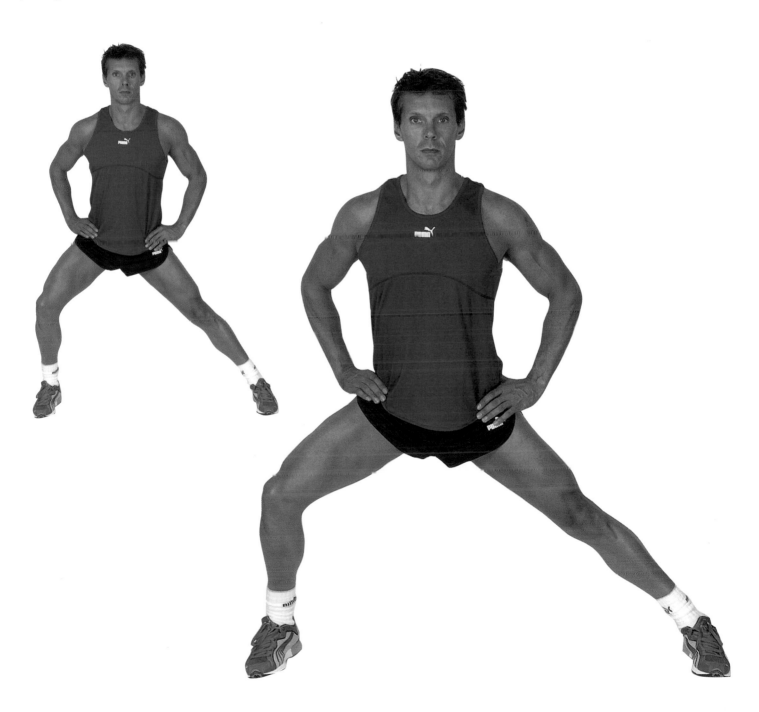

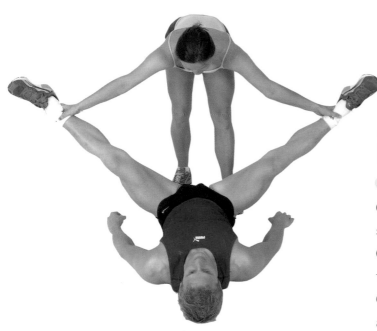

both legs raised **partner**

❶ Lie flat on your back with your hands down toward your sides to help keep your buttocks on the floor.

❷ Raise both feet directly upward, and slowly take them out to the sides.

❸ Your partner will hold the inside of your leg around the ankle joint.

❹ When you reach your maximum stretch without assistance, exhale and have your partner apply light pressure onto your legs to increase the stretch. Relax for a few seconds and repeat to develop the stretch, communicating throughout with your partner.

towel-assisted pull down

❶ Lie on your back, keeping your shoulders and head in contact with the floor.

❷ Use two towels wrapped around your feet to extend the stretch by pulling downward with your hands.

❸ This stretch is best performed with both your heels and buttocks pressed against a wall.

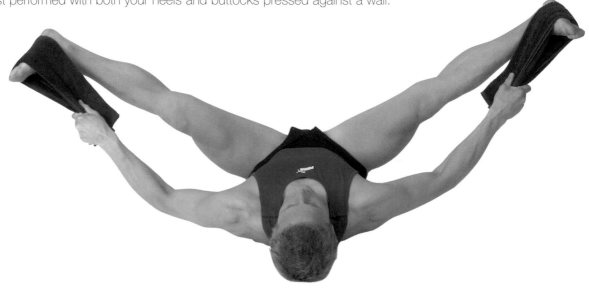

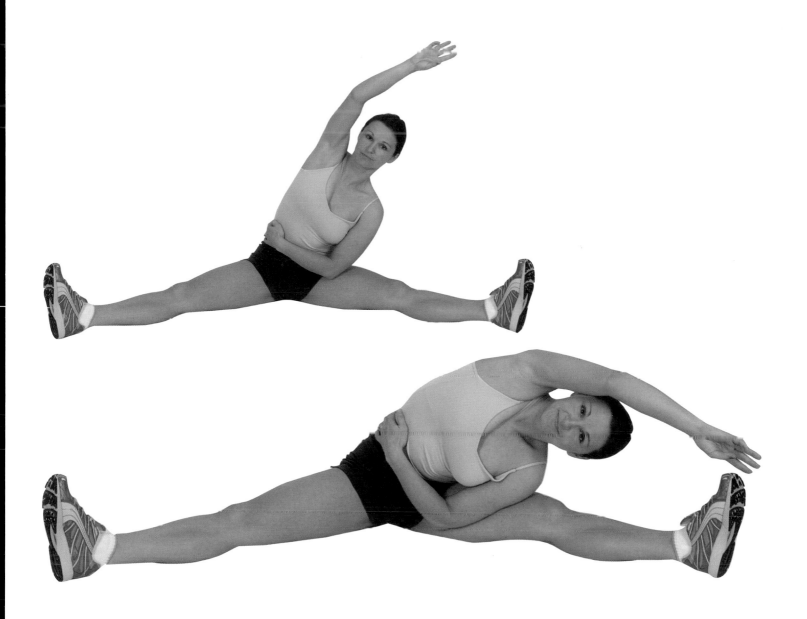

side bend seated

moderate

❶ Sit on the floor with both legs spread wide apart, keeping your heels on the floor.

❷ Extend one arm up over your head and slowly bend from your hip, taking both your arm and the side of your body down toward the opposite leg.

elevated leg

moderate

❶ Stand with one leg resting on a secure, raised surface.

❷ Your back foot should be one stride away with the foot facing outward for greater balance.

❸ Exhale, slowly bending the front leg, taking your pelvis forward.

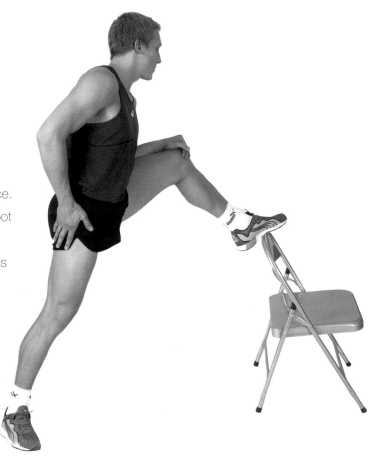

standing leg at right angles

moderate

❶ Rest one heel on a secure raised surface, keeping the foot pointing upward.

❷ Place your other foot firmly on the floor, facing forward.

❸ With your hands grasped overhead, slowly exhale, bending down from your side and taking your head toward the raised knee.

❹ Aim to have the legs at right angles. You may need to bend the leg that is not raised to achieve this.

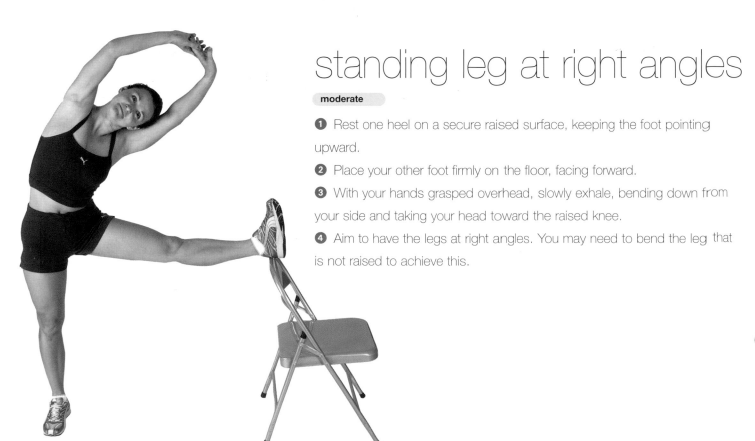

feet together adductors

moderate

❶ Lie on your back, with your heels pulled up toward your groin, keeping the soles of the feet together.

❷ Exhale, slowly applying pressure to the top of the your knees with your hands, pushing the knees downward.

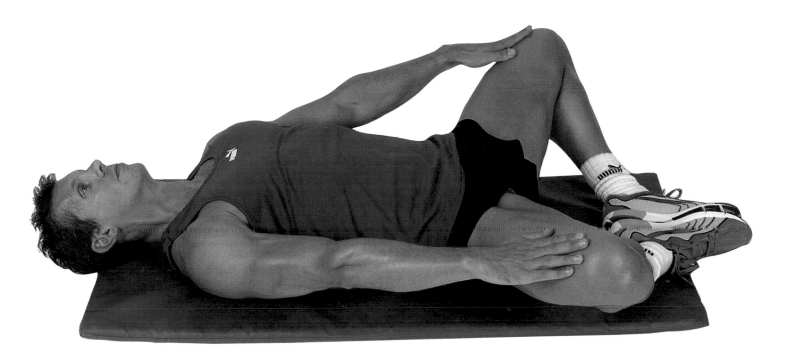

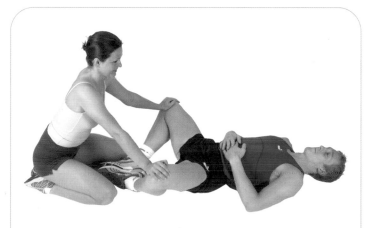

VARIATION: This movement is best performed with a partner pushing down on your knees to increase the stretch.

head to knee **wide leg**

moderate/hard

❶ Sit on the floor with both legs spread wide apart.

❷ While holding one foot, slowly exhale, pulling your head down toward one knee.

❸ Keep the legs straight throughout, using a towel around your foot if necessary.

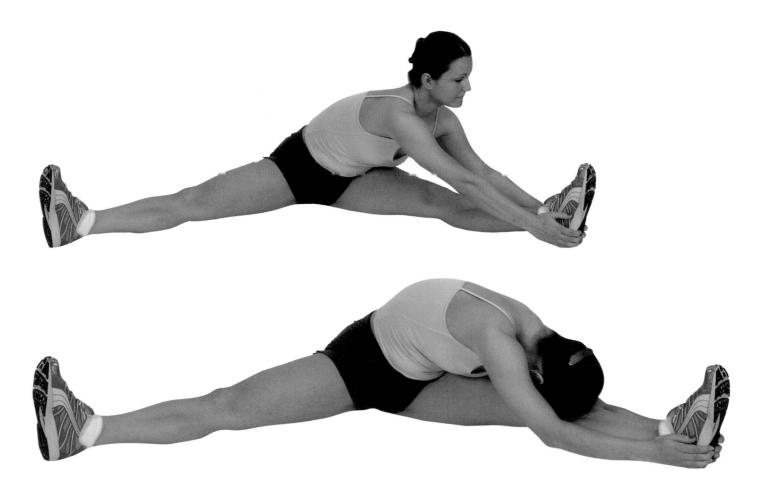

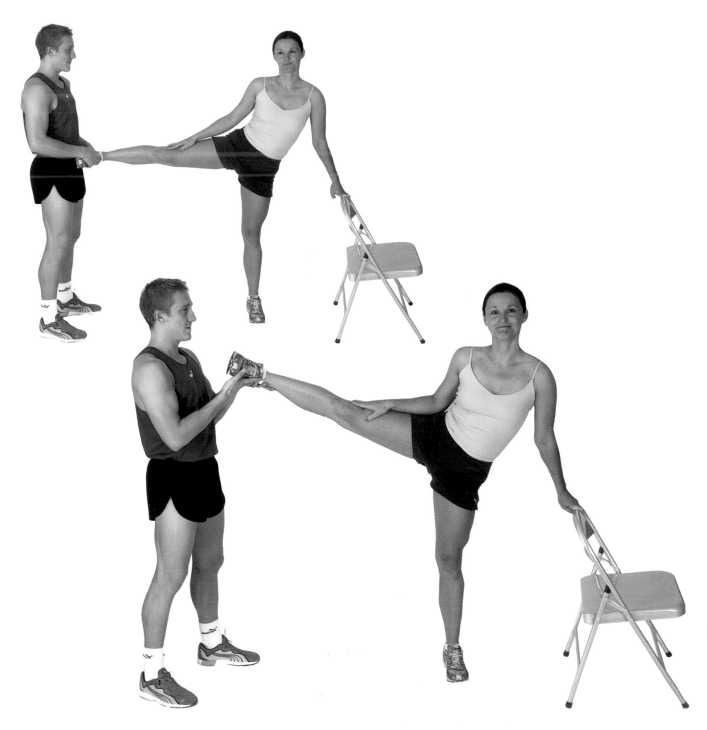

one leg raised

moderate/hard

❶ Balance yourself by holding onto a secure object with both feet facing forward.

❷ Exhale, taking one leg slowly out to the side. Your partner will grab this leg around the inside of the ankle.

❸ On each upward movement, exhale, then rest and inhale for a few seconds, repeating the process.

❹ Avoid forcing the leg up, always controlling the leg as you lower it.

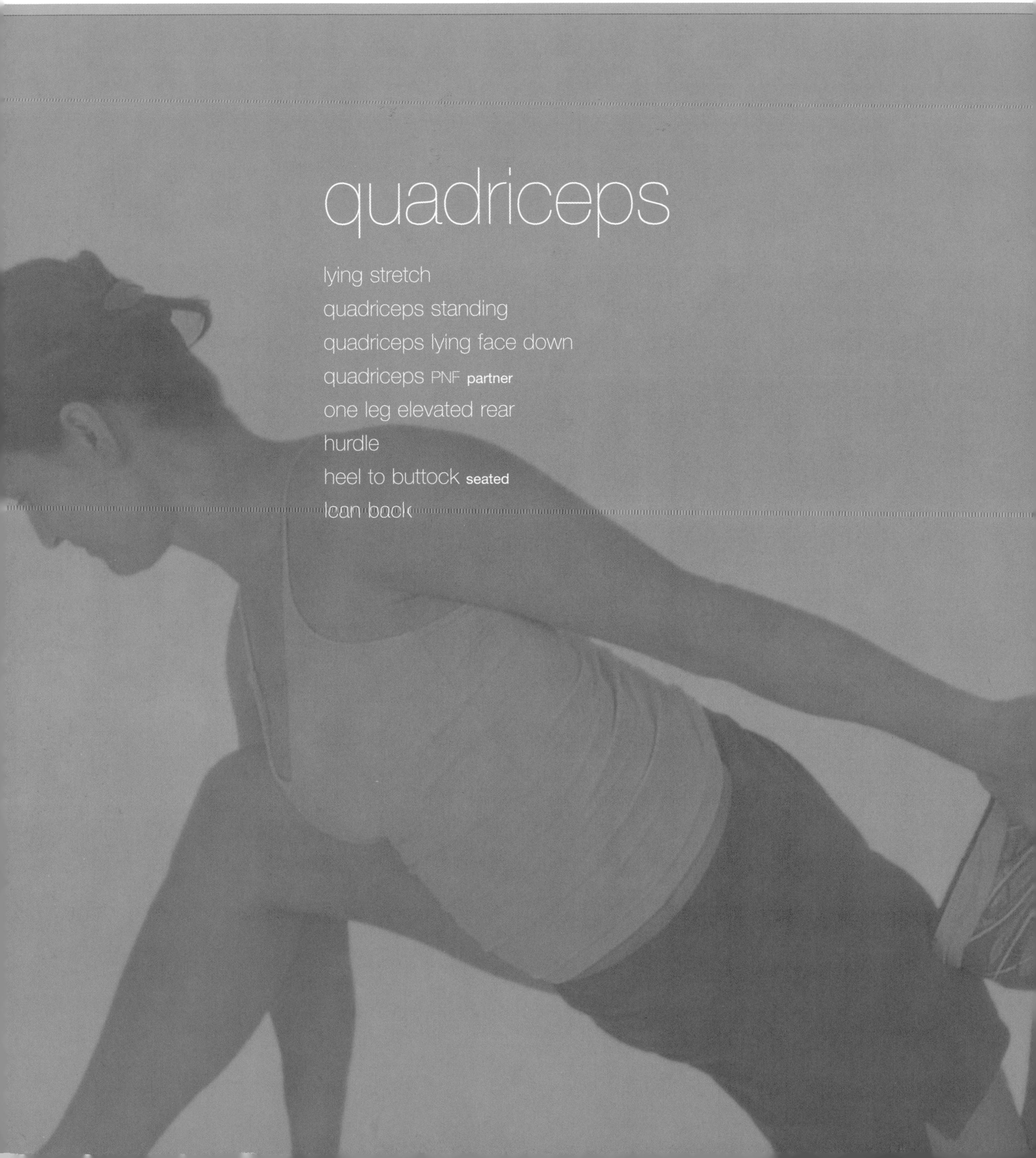

quadriceps

lying stretch

quadriceps standing

quadriceps lying face down

quadriceps PNF **partner**

one leg elevated rear

hurdle

heel to buttock **seated**

lean back

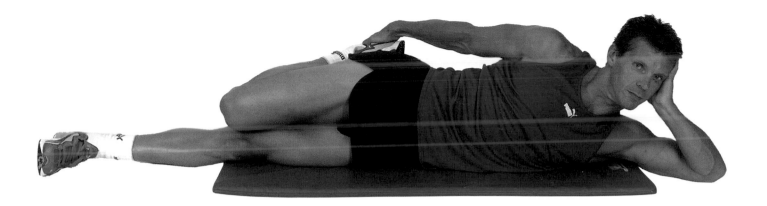

lying stretch

easy

❶ Lie on your side, keeping both the knees and the inside of your thighs together.

❷ Extend the lower leg out straight, keeping the top leg bent and one hand grasping the foot.

❸ Exhale, pulling the foot toward your buttock while you slowly push your pelvis forward.

❹ Use a towel around your foot if you can't reach it.

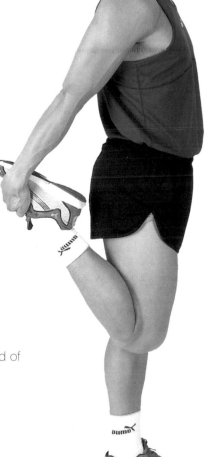

quadriceps standing

easy

❶ Stand holding onto a secure object, or have one hand raised out to the side for balance.

❷ Raise one heel up toward your buttocks, and grasp hold of your foot with one hand.

❸ Inhale, slowly pulling your heel to your buttock while gradually pushing your pelvis forward.

❹ Keep both knees together, having a slight bend in the supporting leg.

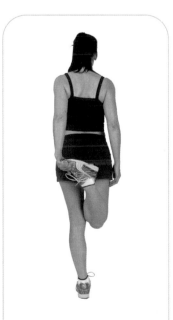

VARIATION: Repeat using the opposite hand to foot.

quadriceps lying face down

easy

❶ Throughout the stretch, concentrate on keeping your knees together. Avoid twisting the pelvis. Keeping your forehead on the floor prevents arching of the lower back.

❷ Gradually pull your heel into your buttock.

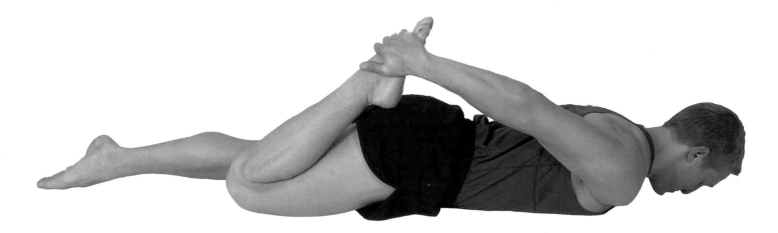

VARIATIONS: Use the opposite arm to leg before being stretched. You may use a towel wrapped around your foot if you can't grab it.

quadriceps PNF **partner**

easy

❶ Lie on your front with your head and elbows resting on the floor.

❷ Bend one leg, which your partner will hold, placing one hand above the ankle joint and the other hand on the sole of the raised foot.

❸ Communicate with your partner as he repeatedly pushes your heel toward your buttocks in small movements, aiming to take and rest the heel on the buttock.

❹ You can also stretch the calf muscle by pushing down on the foot during the stretch.

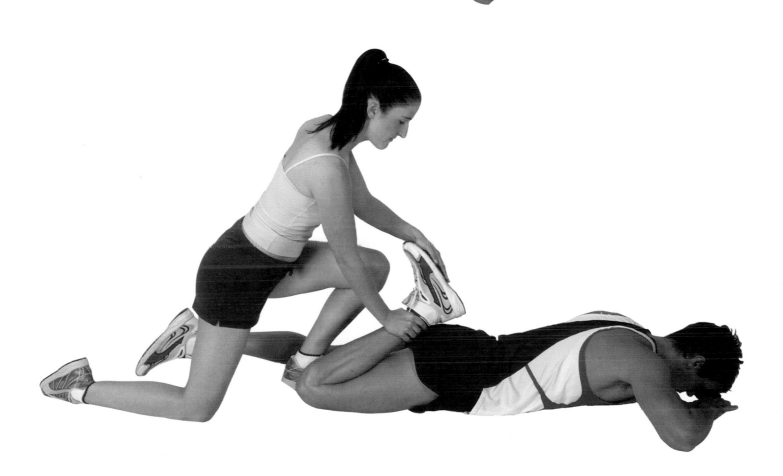

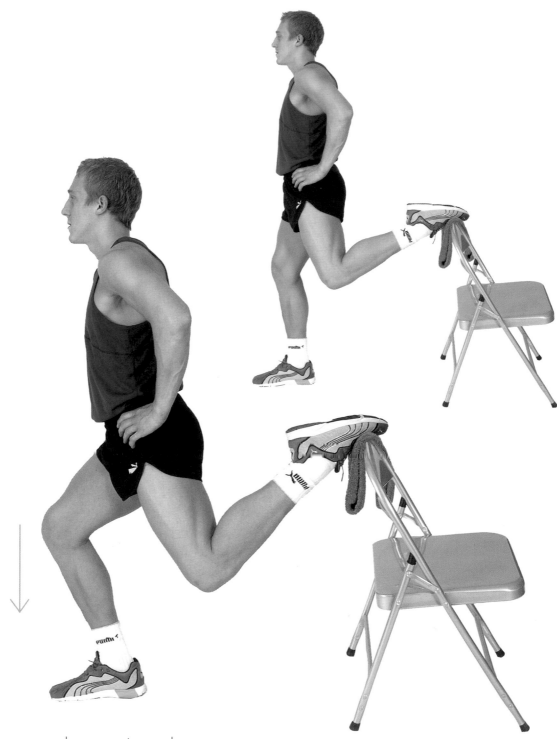

one leg elevated rear

moderate

1. Rest one foot behind you on a secure, raised platform.
2. Extend your front leg one small stride forward, keeping the knee in line with your toes.
3. Inhale, slowly lowering yourself to the floor, keeping your back straight.
4. Hold onto a secure object if you have poor balance.

hurdle

moderate

① Sit on the floor, extending one leg slightly bent out to your front and keeping the other leg bent, with the toes pointing backward and the foot held close to the hip.

② Exhale, lowering your back slowly to the floor and keeping your foot tucked in close to your hip.

③ Increase the stretch by contracting your buttocks while pushing the hips upward.

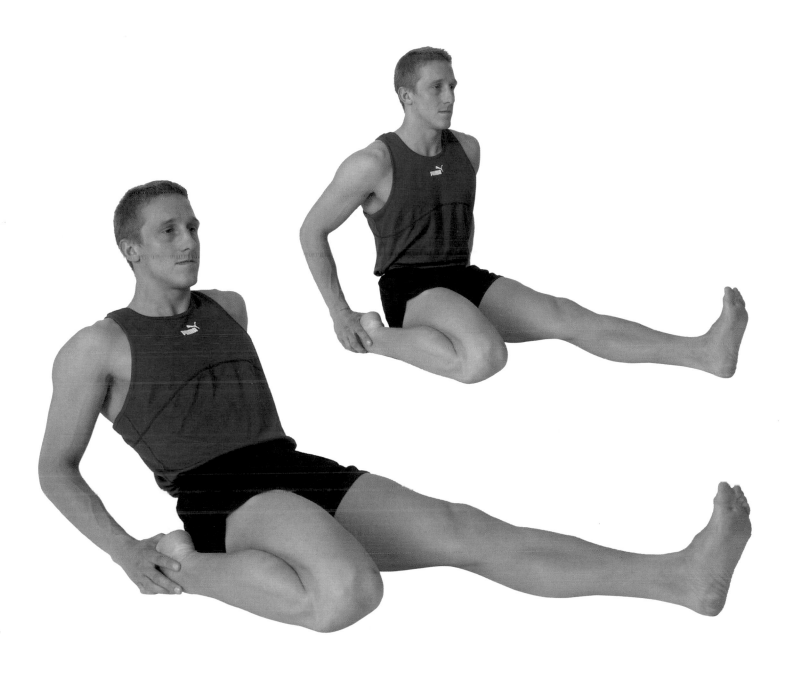

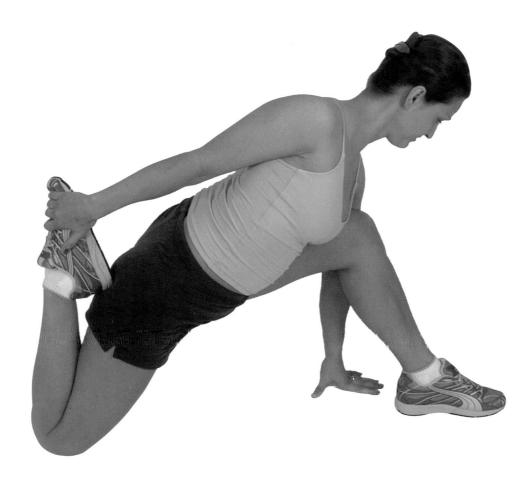

heel to buttock seated

moderate

❶ Rest one knee on the floor, grasping the foot with your hand from the same side.

❷ Extend the other foot and hand out to the front, placing both down firmly for balance.

❸ Keep your ankle, knee, and hip joint aligned while you slowly pull your heel toward your buttock.

lean back

hard

1 Kneel, sitting back on your feet with toes pointing backward, using your hands to fix your feet in place.

2 Exhale slowly while you gradually lower your back to the floor.

3 Concentrate on keeping your knees and lower legs in contact with the floor.

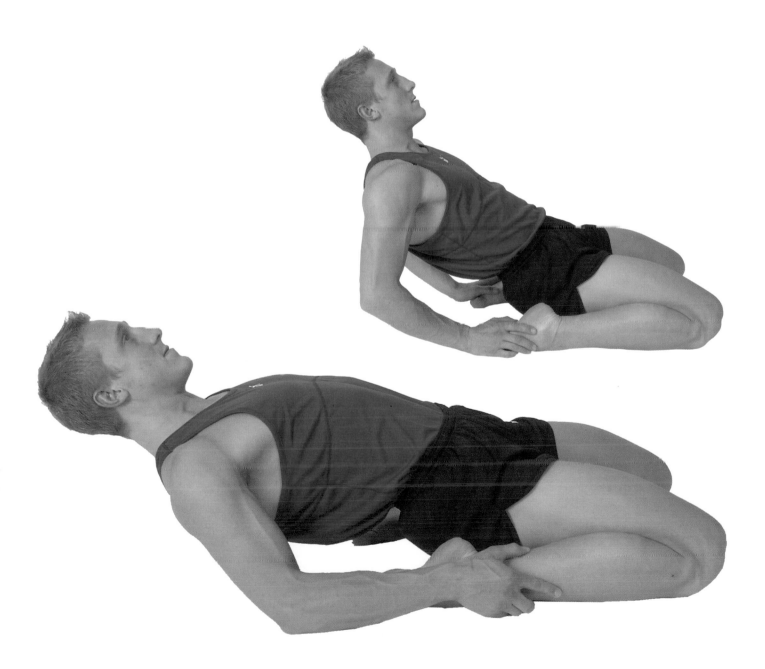

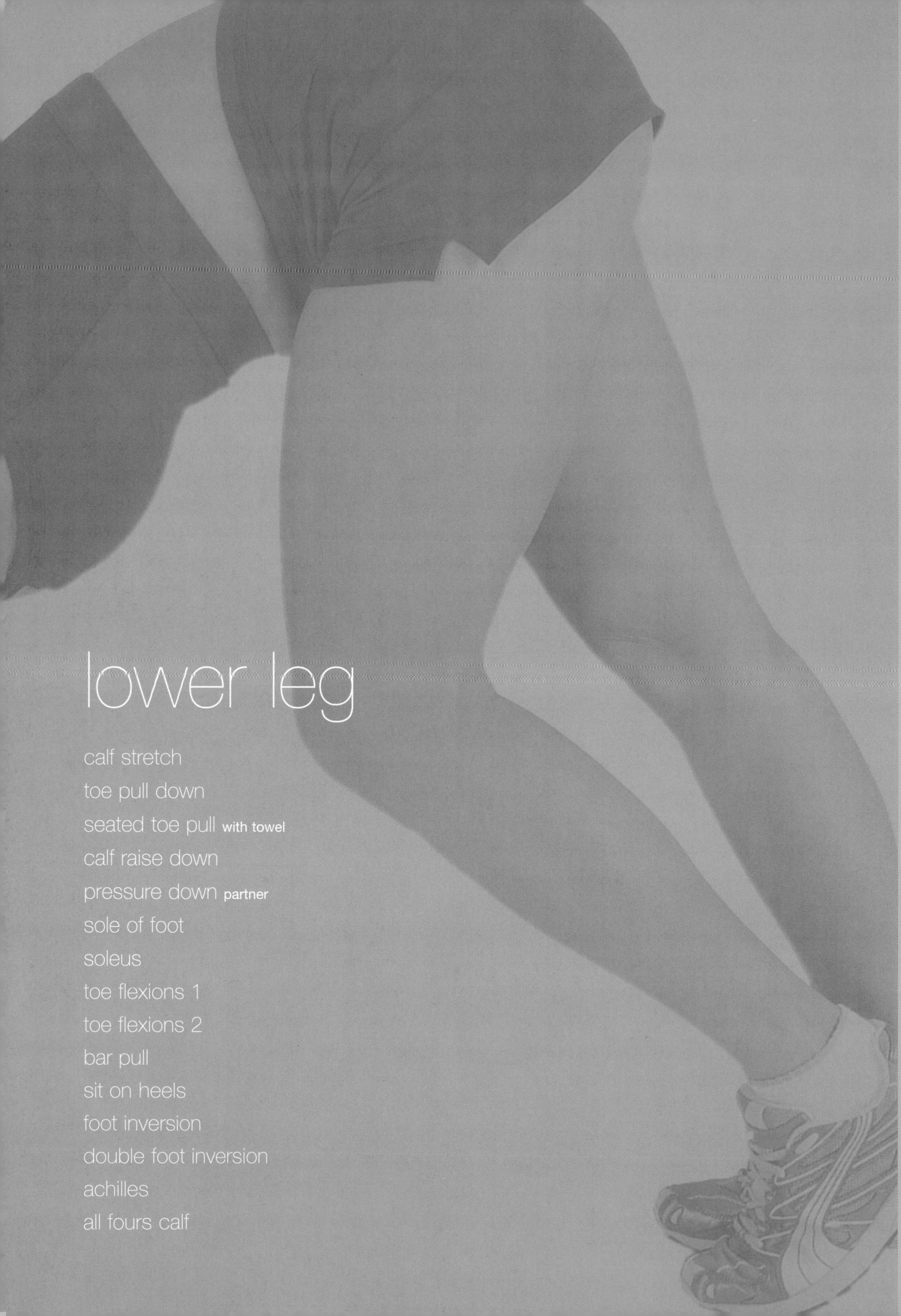

lower leg

calf stretch

toe pull down

seated toe pull **with towel**

calf raise down

pressure down **partner**

sole of foot

soleus

toe flexions 1

toe flexions 2

bar pull

sit on heels

foot inversion

double foot inversion

achilles

all fours calf

calf stretch

easy

❶ Feet should be a shoulder width apart. You can confirm this by performing the stretch by standing on either side of a straight line on the floor.

❷ When you take your rear foot back, it should not cross or move away from the midline. Your foot should be pointing forward with your heel either flat on the floor or raised if aiming to develop the stretch.

❸ Your front leg should bend so that when you look down over your knee, you can see the tip of your toes. Lean forward, keeping a straight line with your heel, hip, and head. This stretch is best performed against a wall.

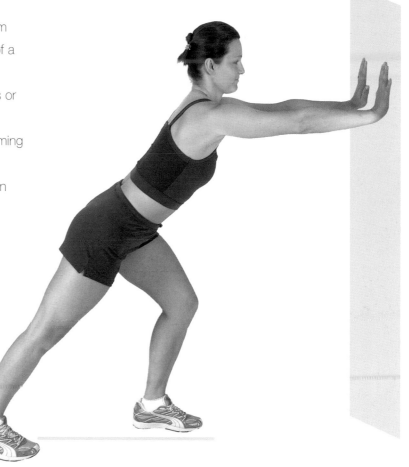

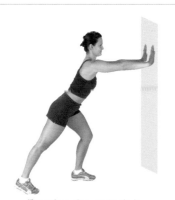

VARIATIONS: Develop the stretch by beginning with your heel raised on your rear foot, stretching the calf. Relax, take a deep breath, and then stretch again, exhaling slowly.

toe pull down

easy

❶ Cross one leg over the opposite knee.

❷ Slowly pull the toes downward by applying pressure from your fingers on the top of your toes while your thumb pushes upward against the ball of your foot.

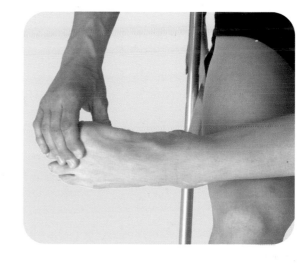

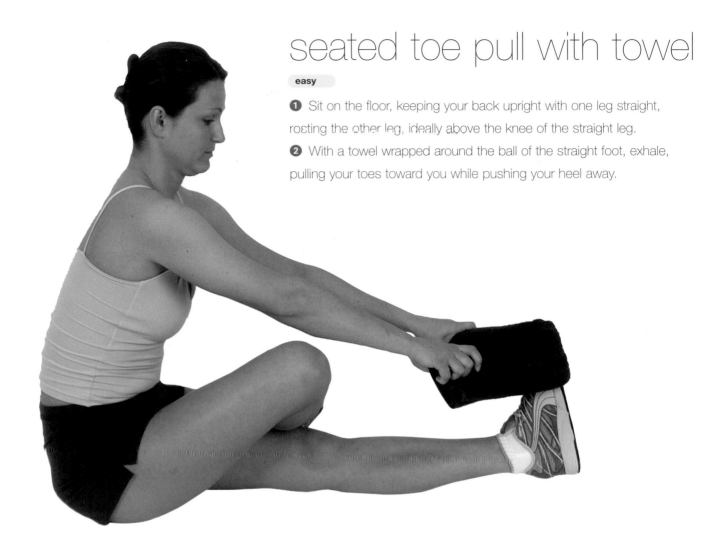

seated toe pull with towel

easy

❶ Sit on the floor, keeping your back upright with one leg straight, resting the other leg, ideally above the knee of the straight leg.

❷ With a towel wrapped around the ball of the straight foot, exhale, pulling your toes toward you while pushing your heel away.

calf raise down

easy

❶ Stand on a raised platform on the balls of your feet, holding onto a secure object for balance.

❷ Exhale, slowly dropping your heels down toward the floor and allowing your feet to raise naturally.

This movement can be performed using either one or both feet.

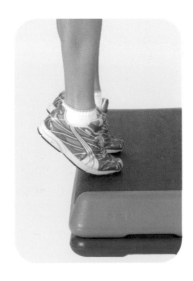
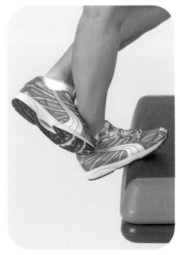

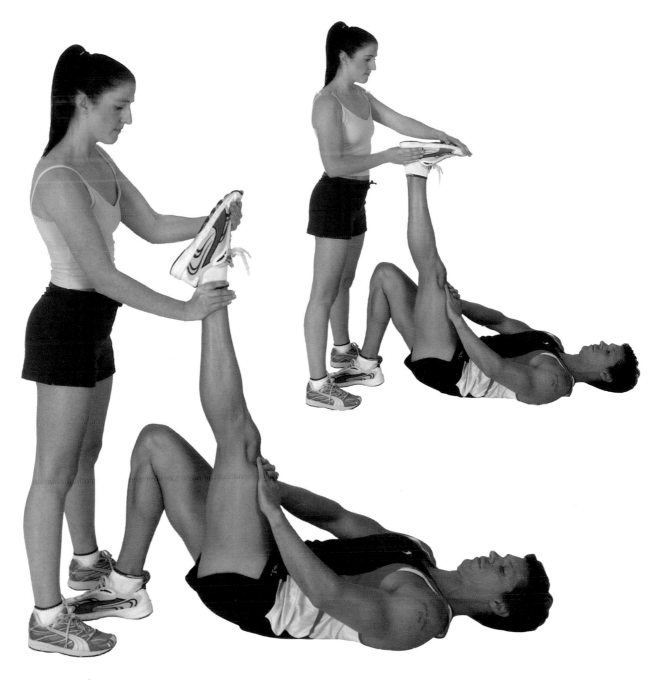

pressure down **partner**

easy

❶ Lie on your back with one leg extended straight up, keeping your other leg bent and your foot flat on the floor close to your buttocks.

❷ Your partner will hold the leg straight with one hand around your heel while applying downward pressure on the ball of your foot, bending it toward your knee.

❸ While in the same position, your partner can also pull your foot upward by placing one hand on the front of your foot and pulling upward, using the other hand to fix the heel in place.

❹ Communicate with your partner and keep your hands on the thigh of the raised leg to fix it upright.

sole of foot

easy

❶ Kneel on all fours with the tips of your toes in contact with the floor just beneath your buttocks.

❷ Exhale, pushing your buttocks backward while placing the balls of your feet on the floor, bringing your heels up to your buttocks.

Avoid wearing shoes for this stretch.

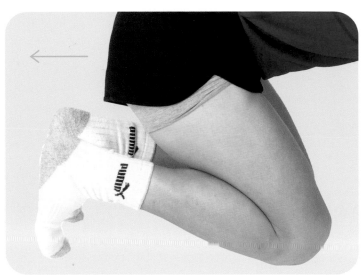

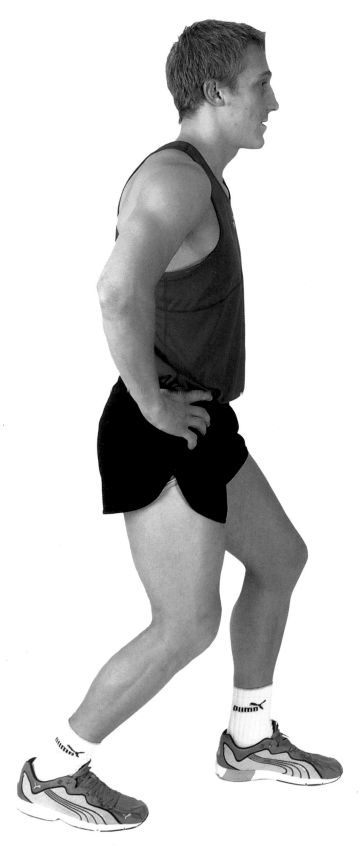

soleus

easy

❶ Stand with both feet flat on the floor, pointing forward, half a stride apart.

❷ Keeping your back straight, with your hands on your hips, exhale and lower yourself down, resting your body weight on the rear foot.

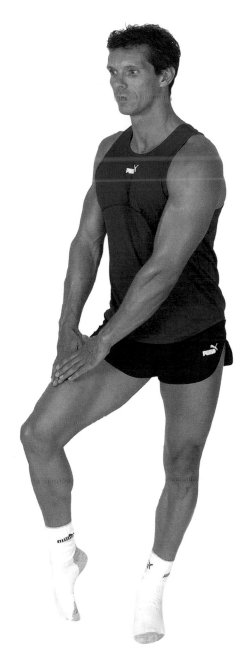

toe flexions 1

easy

❶ Stand with one leg bent, resting the toenails on the floor and keeping the heel raised.

❷ Exhale, gently pressing downward and forward with your toes, making an arch with the foot by dropping the heel toward the floor while keeping the toes in contact with the floor.

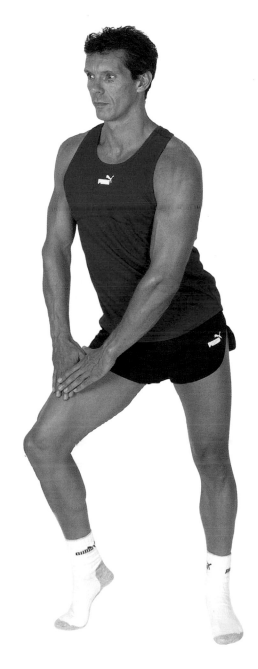

toe flexions 2

easy

❶ Stand with one leg bent, keeping your toes and the ball of your foot in contact with the floor.

❷ Exhale slowly, pushing down on your toes while lifting the heel of your foot.

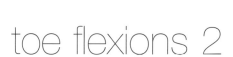

bar pull

easy/moderate

❶ Hold a secure object with both hands together at waist height.

❷ Keeping your hands fixed, slowly take your feet backward, keeping them shoulder width apart, toes pointing toward your hands with your feet flat on the floor.

❸ Exhale, extending your buttocks backward, keeping your arms and legs straight.

❹ Repeat again, pointing your feet toward each other.

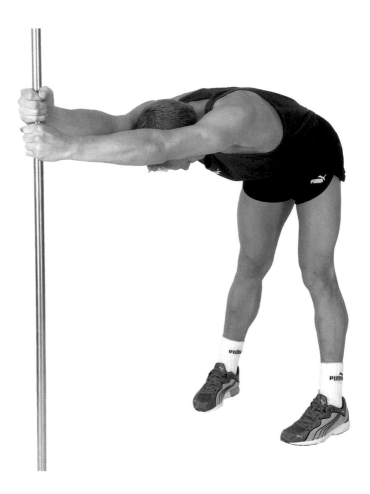

sit on heels

moderate

❶ Elevate your feet with a rolled towel and then slowly sit your buttocks back onto your heels.

❷ Concentrate on keeping your knees and ankles together with your feet pointing directly behind you.

❸ While in this position, you can pull upward on your toes to increase the stretch along your shin.

Avoid this stretch if you have knee problems.

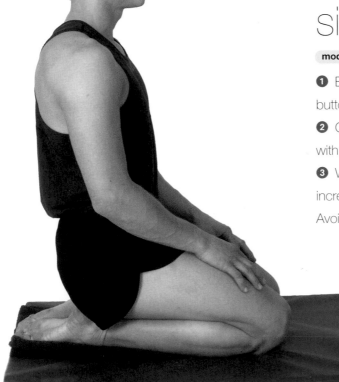

foot inversion

easy/moderate

❶ Extend one leg forward, keeping it as straight as possible.

❷ Apply pressure on the outside of the foot, aiming to turn your outer foot inward.

double foot inversion

moderate/hard

❶ Slowly lean forward from the hips, aiming to hold each foot with both legs straight.

❷ Exhale, gradually turning your feet inward, using your hands to apply sufficient pressure.

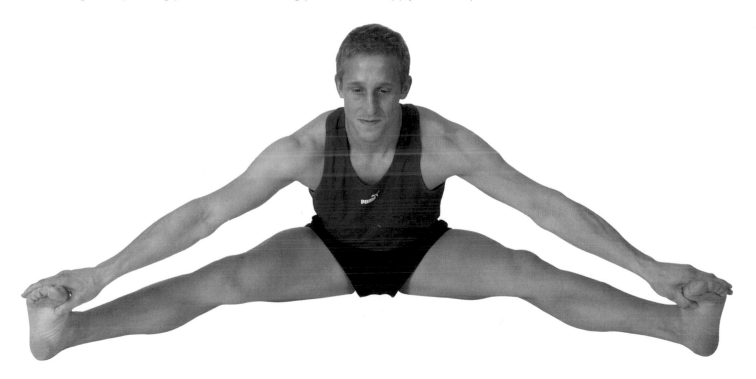

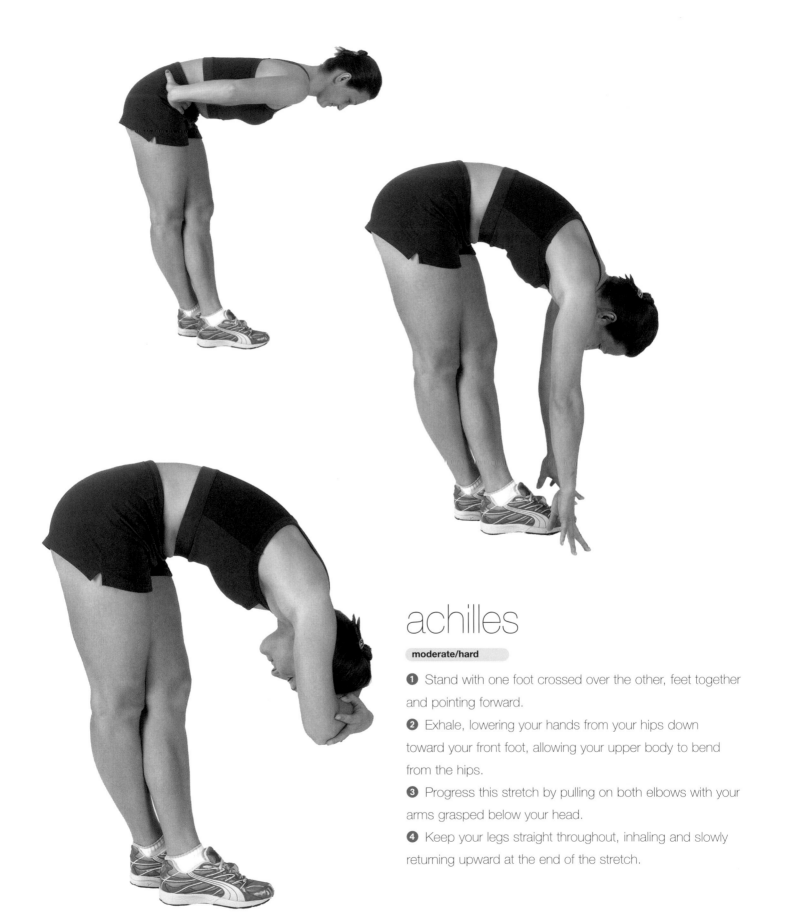

achilles

moderate/hard

❶ Stand with one foot crossed over the other, feet together and pointing forward.

❷ Exhale, lowering your hands from your hips down toward your front foot, allowing your upper body to bend from the hips.

❸ Progress this stretch by pulling on both elbows with your arms grasped below your head.

❹ Keep your legs straight throughout, inhaling and slowly returning upward at the end of the stretch.

all fours calf

moderate/hard

1 Slowly lean forward, placing both hands flat on the floor, one large stride away, and bending your legs if necessary.

2 Exhale slowly, straightening one leg and placing the heel down to the floor.

3 Inhale, then repeat the stretch on the opposite leg, this time pushing down on your toes with the heel raised slightly off the floor.

> **VARIATIONS:** Resting your hands on a raised platform will release the tension in your hamstrings.

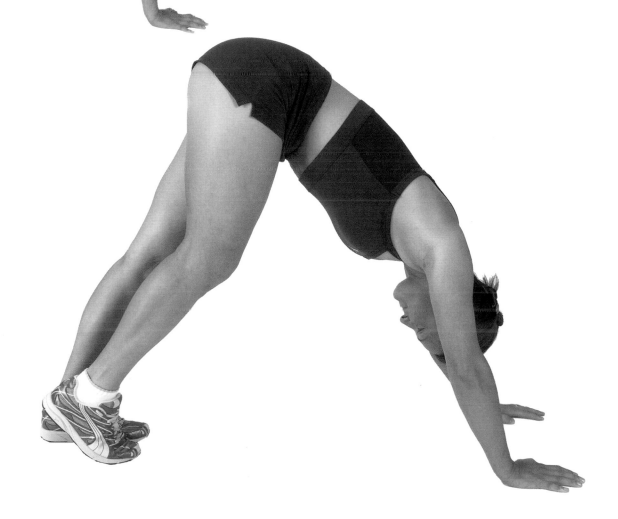

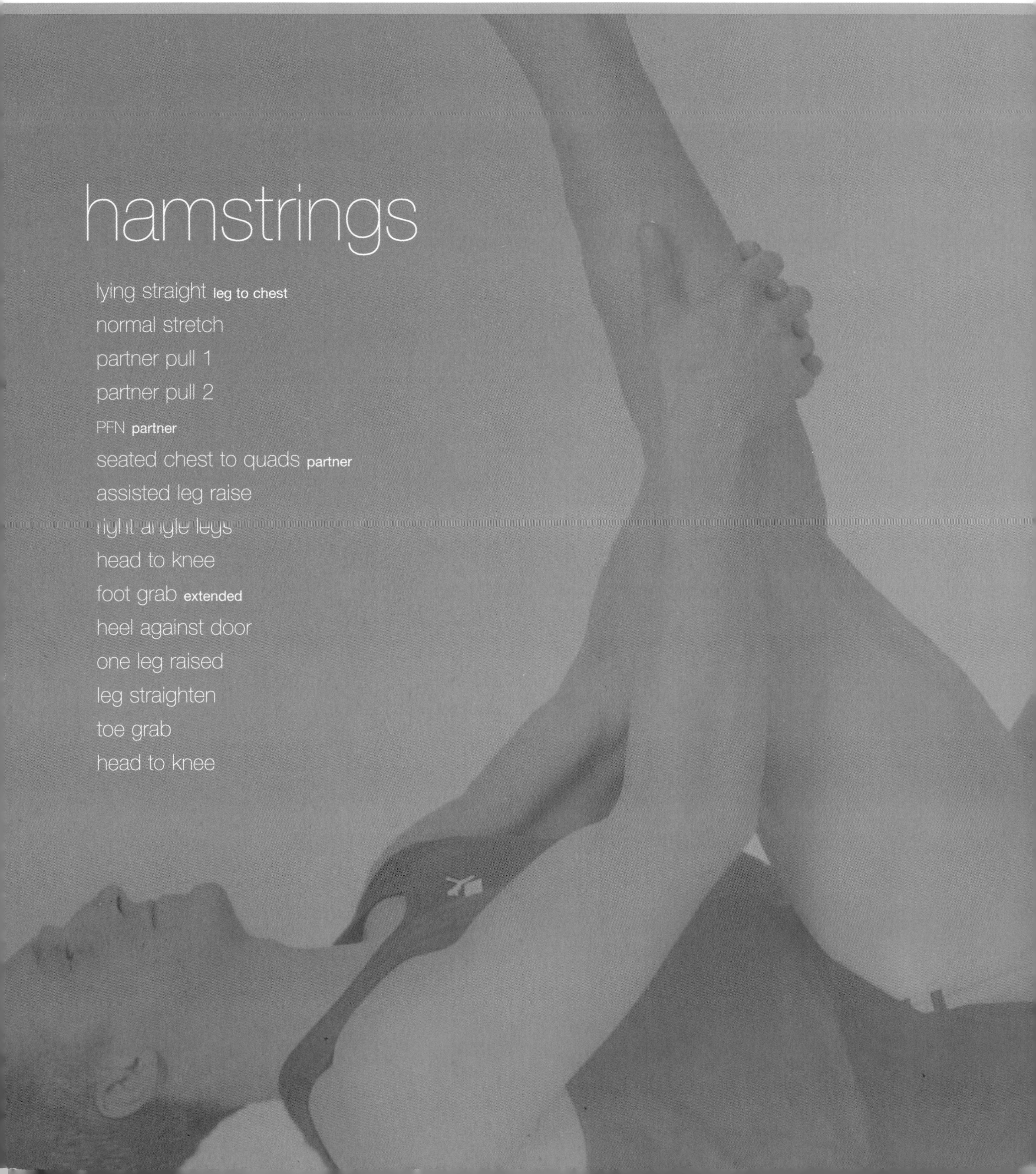

hamstrings

lying straight **leg to chest**

normal stretch

partner pull 1

partner pull 2

PFN **partner**

seated chest to quads **partner**

assisted leg raise

right angle legs

head to knee

foot grab **extended**

heel against door

one leg raised

leg straighten

toe grab

head to knee

lying straight leg to chest

easy

❶ Lie comfortably on your back, concentrating on keeping both your head and buttocks in contact with the floor.

❷ Slowly extend one leg upward, grasping it with both hands either around the calf, the hamstrings, or a combination of both.

❸ Pull your leg toward your chest, keeping it straight. When the tension builds up in your hamstrings, relax the stretch a little by contracting your quadriceps on the same leg.

❹ If necessary, use a towel wrapped around your foot in order to keep your head on the floor.

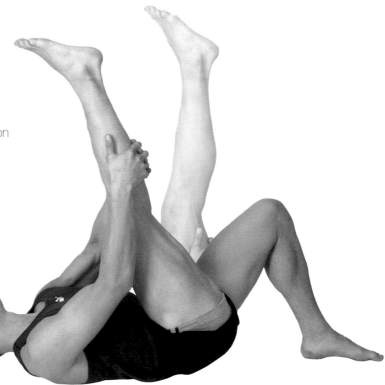

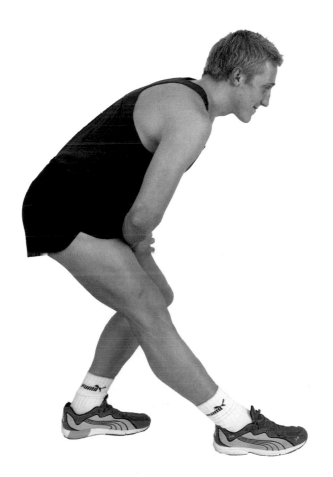

normal stretch

easy

❶ Stand with your feet shoulder width apart, one foot extended half a step forward.

❷ Keeping the front leg straight, bend your rear leg, resting both hands on the bent thigh.

❸ Slowly exhale, tilting both buttocks upward, keeping the front leg straight and both feet flat on the floor, pointing forward.

❹ Inhale slowly and relax from the stretch. Repeat the stretch again, this time beginning with the toes of the front foot raised toward the ceiling but keeping the heel on the floor.

partner pull 1

easy

❶ Sit on the floor with your legs straight, facing your partner and pushing the soles of your feet against his feet.

❷ Both partners need to hold one end of a towel, keeping their arms straight and parallel with the floor.

❸ Communicate with your partner, as one of you leans back, pulling on the towel while the other bends forward from the hip.

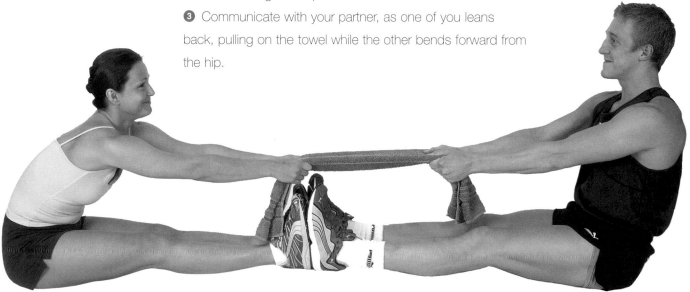

partner pull 2

moderate

❶ Sit on the floor, facing your partner.

❷ Bend one leg so that your foot rests on the inside of your thigh while your other leg is straight, resting against the upper shin of your partner's leg, as he adopts the same position.

❸ While grasping each other's wrists, communicate with each other as you exhale and bend forward, as your partner leans back, bringing your chest down to the knee of the extended leg.

❹ Perform the stretch using a controlled movement, keeping your feet, legs, and buttocks in contact with the floor.

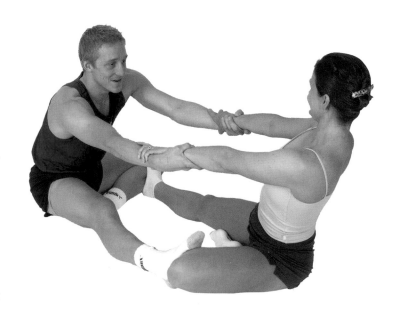

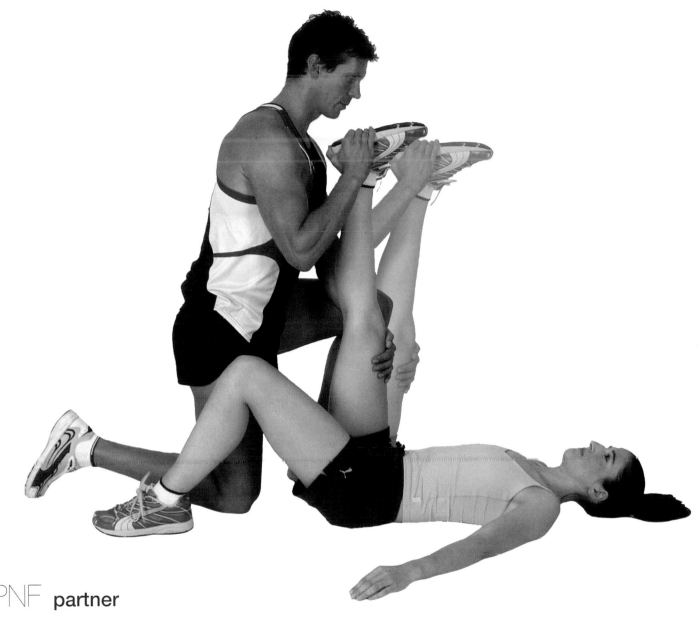

PNF partner

easy/moderate

❶ Lie on your back with both arms out to the side, head on the floor, and one foot flat on the floor close to your buttock.

❷ Raise the other leg straight with your partner grasping the heel and front of the thigh.

❸ Communicate with your partner as he pushes your leg toward you as you push your heel toward him.

❹ If your partner is weak, rest your heel against his shoulder, so he can lean forward to increase the stretch.

❺ Avoid applying too much force and perform the stretch in a sequence. Push for ten to fifteen seconds, then relax for five seconds, before repeating another two to three times, increasing the range of the stretch each time.

❻ Concentrate on keeping your buttocks firmly on the floor, contracting your quadriceps to help relax the hamstrings.

seated chest to quads **partner**

moderate

1 Sit on the floor with one leg straight, toes pointing upward, and the other leg bent, either behind (hurdle position) or resting against the opposite inner thigh.

2 Exhale, extending both hands toward the upright foot on the straight leg.

3 Communicate with your partner as he aids you with the stretch by applying pressure to your upper back.

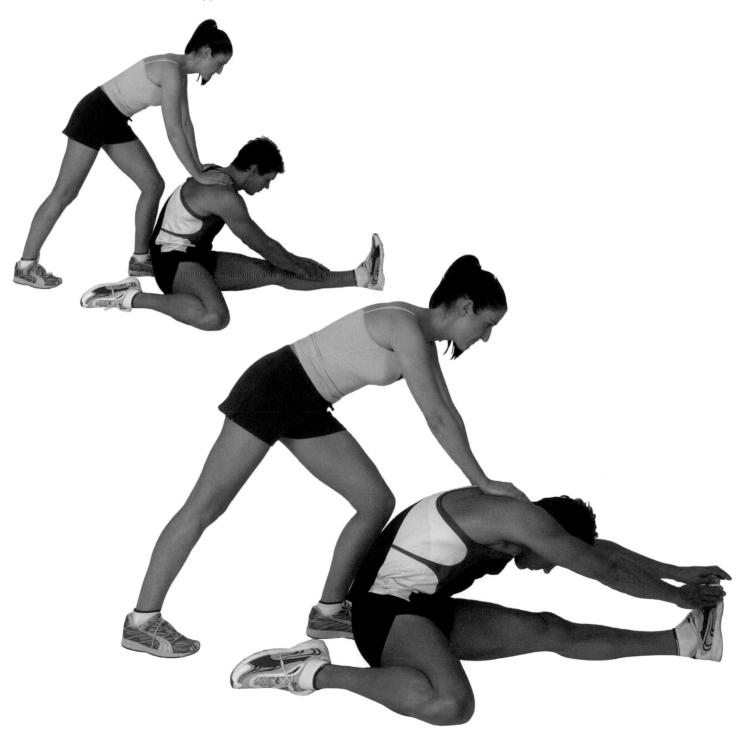

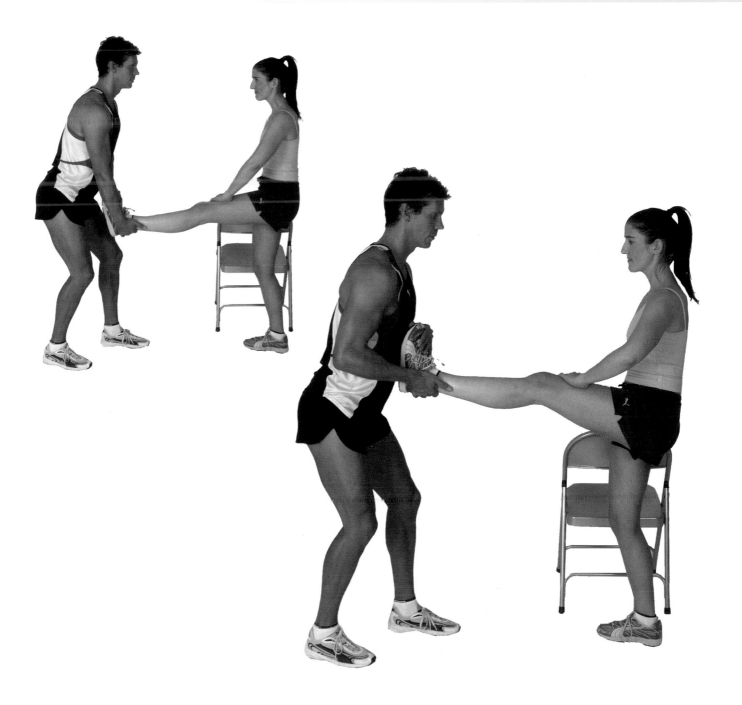

assisted leg raise

moderate

❶ Hold a secure object for balance and raise one leg, which your partner will hold at the heel and foot, keeping your toes pointing upward.

❷ Place your other hand on the raised thigh to help keep that leg straight. The supporting leg should be slightly bent.

❸ Exhale slowly while your partner gently raises your leg.

❹ Contract your quadriceps to help relax your hamstrings and increase the stretch.

❺ Develop the stretch by relaxing for a few seconds before repeating two to three times.

right angle legs

hard

❶ Sit on the floor, extending one hand out to the side and rear for balance.

❷ Use the other hand to grab the heel of the foot on the same side.

❸ Slowly exhale, bringing the leg up toward your shoulder.

❹ Keep the leg straight throughout the stretch and avoid letting it go out to the side or across your body.

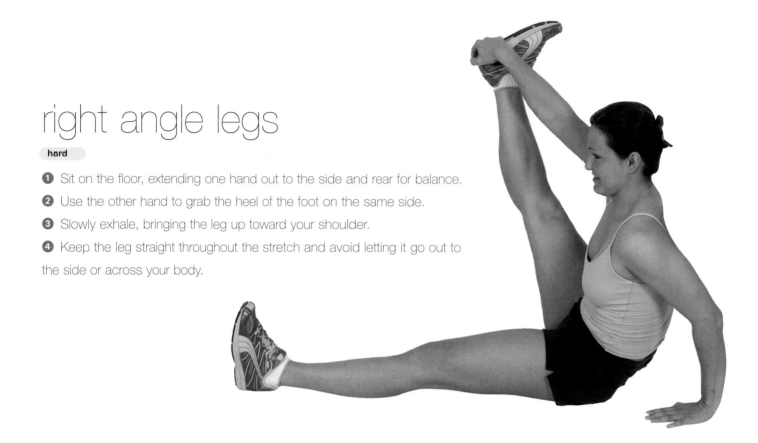

head to knee

moderate/hard

❶ Sit on the floor with both legs apart.

❷ Keep one leg straight, foot pointing upward, and the other leg bent, foot firmly on the floor.

❸ Grasp each leg with one hand in order to fix the leg position.

❹ Exhale slowly, aiming to rest your head on the knee of the straight leg.

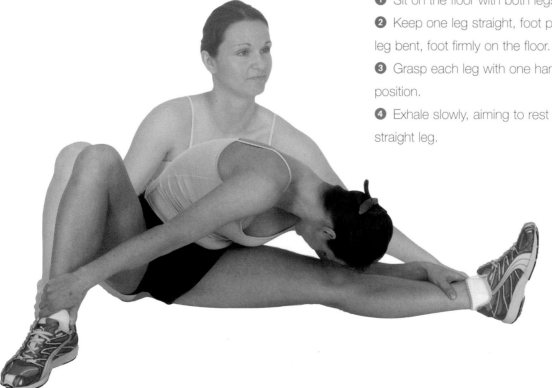

foot grab **extended**

`moderate`

1 You can work into this stretch by slowly sliding the heel along the floor. As you feel the tension behind your knee and hamstrings, contract the quadriceps to relax the opposing muscle.

2 This stretch can be performed with either one or both feet and also with the aid of a towel wrapped around the ball of your feet if you're unable to straighten the leg while holding onto your feet.

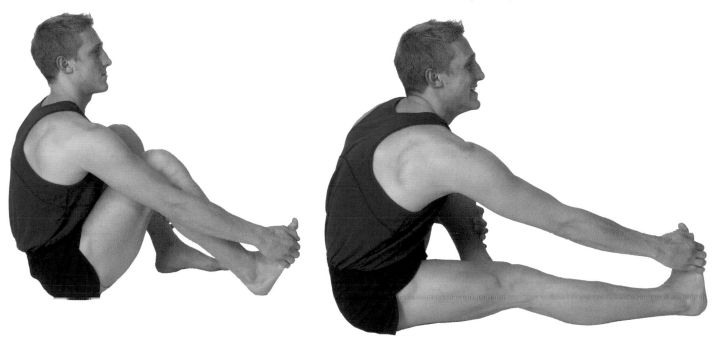

heel against door

`moderate`

1 Lie on your back, either in a doorway or at the corner of a wall, keeping both buttocks in front of the wall line.

2 Rest both hands down by your sides, with the leg furthest from the wall extended straight and the heel of the other foot resting raised up against the wall.

3 Slowly contract the quadriceps of the raised foot, bringing both hips forward toward the wall line and bringing the raised foot closer toward your head, keeping the leg straight.

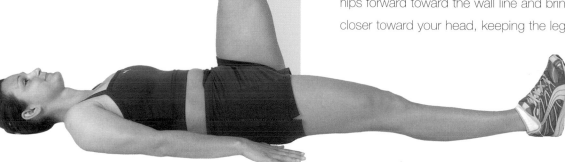

one leg raised

easy/moderate

1 Stand one leg width away from a secure raised platform.

2 Rest the heel of one leg on the platform, or if using a chair, rest your ankle on a folded towel.

3 Keeping your raised leg straight, exhale, sliding your hands down the raised leg and aiming to bring your chest to your knee.

4 You can increase the stretch by bending your supporting leg, taking your buttocks toward the floor, and keeping your pelvis facing forward.

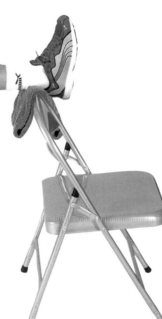

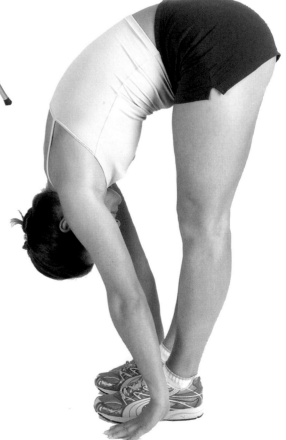

leg straighten

hard

1 Place one foot half a stride in front of you, keeping both feet facing forward, shoulder width apart, legs straight.

2 Exhale, slowly lowering both of your hands toward the floor of your front leg.

3 Initiate the movement with front foot raised, heel on the floor, with rear leg bent. Aim to place the front foot firmly on the floor and straighten the rear leg.

4 Avoid bouncing during the stretch. Contract the quadriceps to help relax the hamstring muscles.

toe grab

moderate/hard

❶ Stand with feet and knees together, keeping your legs straight.

❷ Exhale and slowly bend forward from your hips, taking both hands toward your feet.

❸ Progress this stretch by pulling up on your toes while extending your buttocks upward.

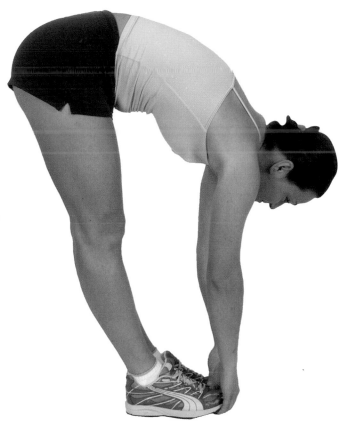

head to knee

hard

❶ Sit on the floor with both legs extended straight to the front, feet pointing upward, knees and ankles together.

❷ Exhale, grasping your ankles with both hands, and gently pull your head down toward your knees. Wrap a towel around your feet if you are unable to reach your ankles.

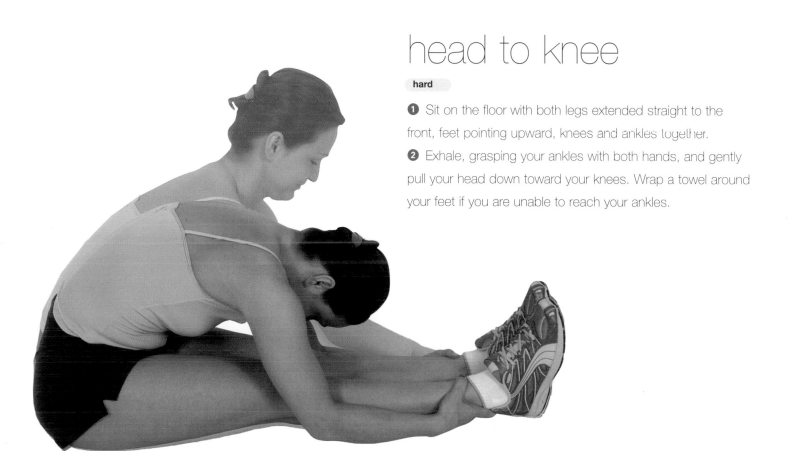

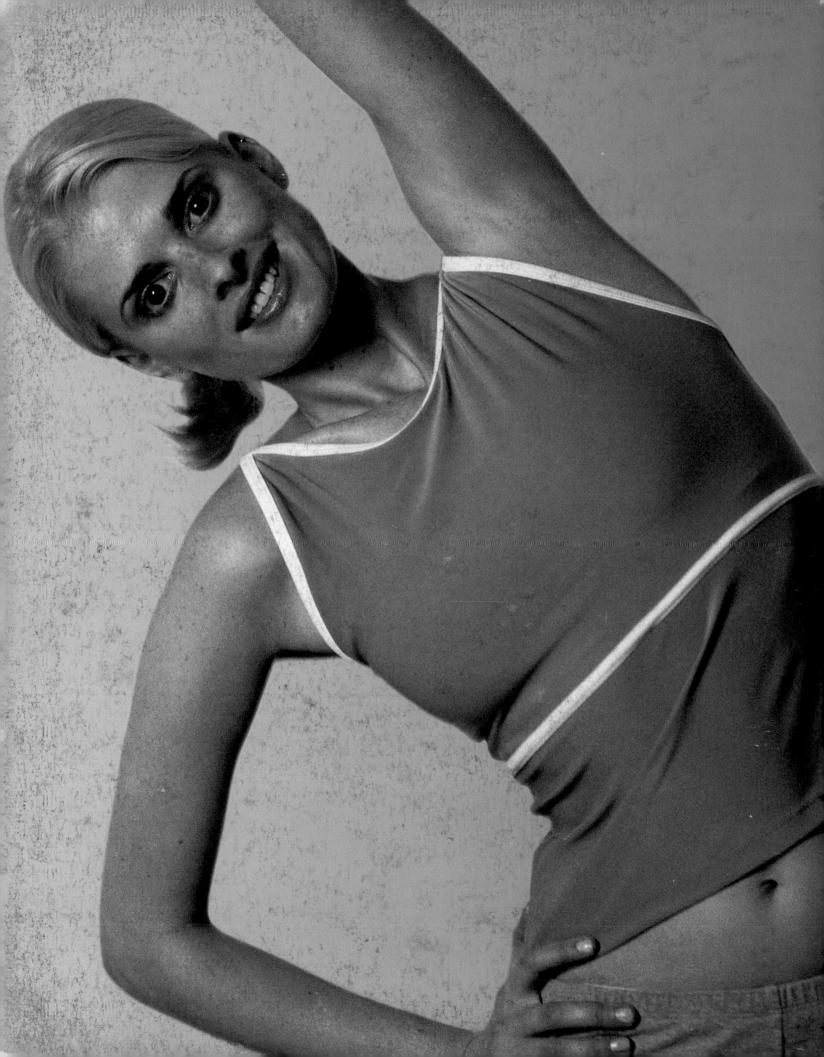

stretch programs
for specific sports

dynamic stretching

dynamic stretching

Dynamic stretching involves a series of gentle, controlled movements that are designed to warm up your body before embarking on an exercise routine. The emphasis is on gradually increasing the speed and reach of your movements, taking you to the limit of your range but — crucially — not attempting to force you beyond what your body can do. Most of us indulge in dynamic stretching each day without even realizing it. When you get out of bed and slowly stretch your limbs, you're effectively warming your body up for the rest of the day.

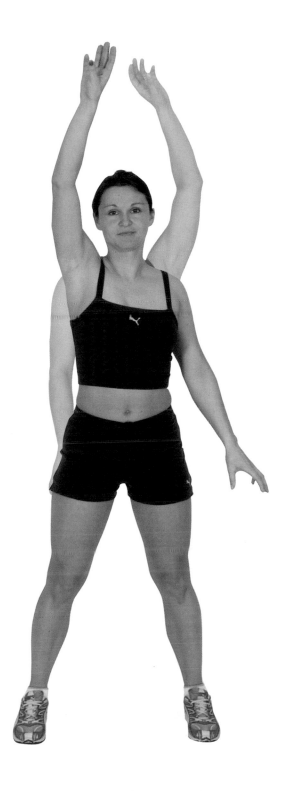

backstroke

❶ Stand upright with your feet wide apart and facing forward.

❷ Begin by taking one hand at a time up over your head in a complete circle, bringing the hand close to your hip on the downward phase of the circle.

❸ Gradually build up the speed, keeping your arms straight and fingers pointed.

❹ Progress to taking both arms back at the same time—your arms will not be able to pass so close to your hips during the downward phase here.

Work for one to three minutes.

breaststroke

❶ Stand with your legs shoulder width apart, bending forward from the hips, with your head facing down, eyes directed forward slightly.

❷ Perform small breaststroke movements, keeping your elbows high as you extend your arms out in large, smooth movements.

Work for one minute.

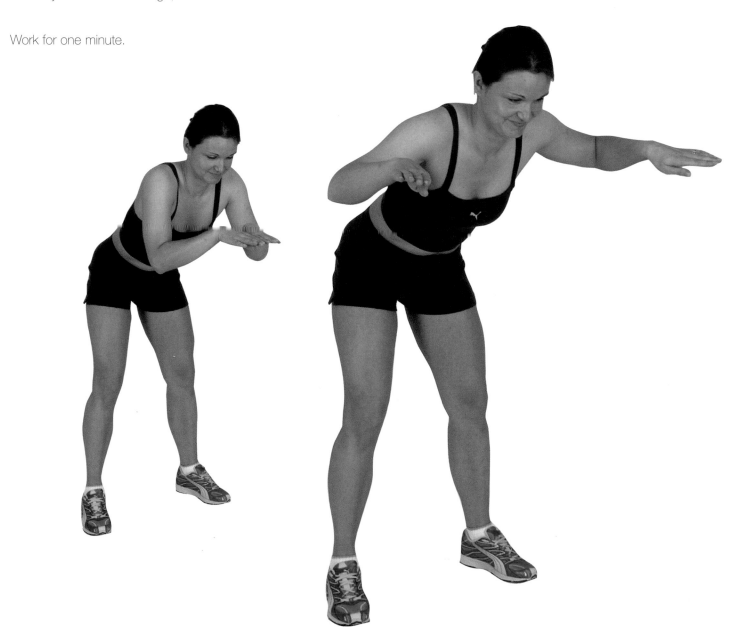

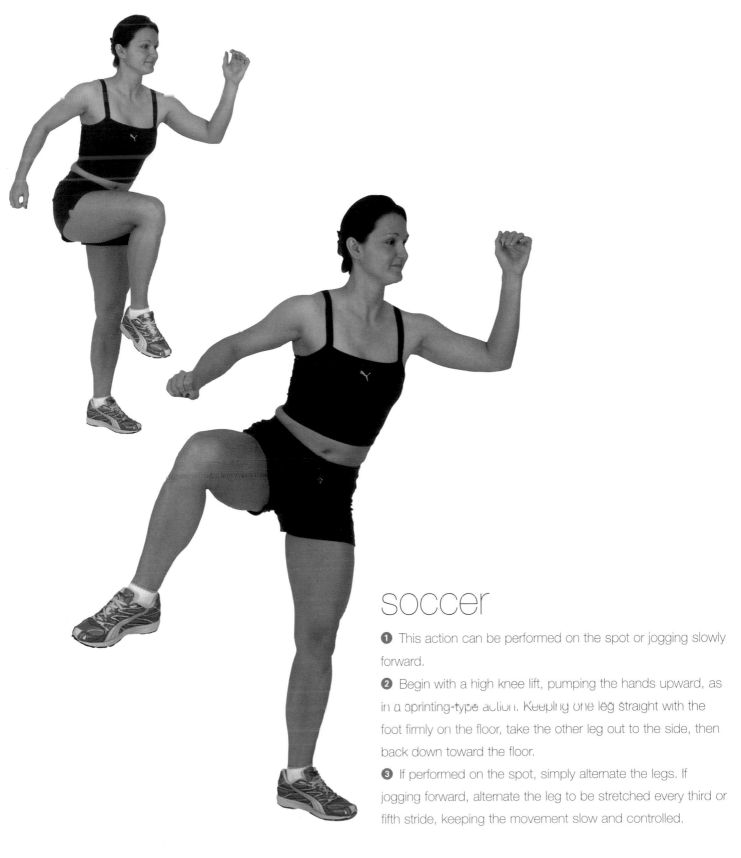

soccer

1 This action can be performed on the spot or jogging slowly forward.

2 Begin with a high knee lift, pumping the hands upward, as in a sprinting-type action. Keeping one leg straight with the foot firmly on the floor, take the other leg out to the side, then back down toward the floor.

3 If performed on the spot, simply alternate the legs. If jogging forward, alternate the leg to be stretched every third or fifth stride, keeping the movement slow and controlled.

Work for two to four minutes.

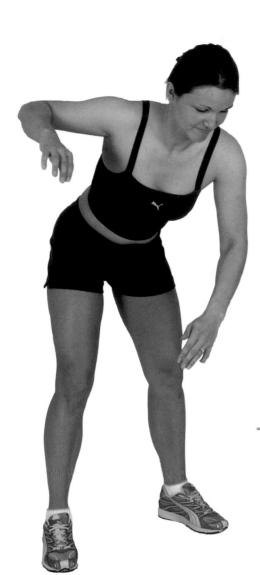

front crawl

❶ Stand with feet shoulder width apart, leaning forward from the waist and looking down in front of you.

❷ Keeping your arms bent, extend alternate hands forward to your midline, and then back to the side of your hips.

❸ Concentrate on keeping the movements small at first, gradually increasing the size of the stretch while steadily building up speed. Remember to use smooth, controlled actions throughout.

❹ Avoid rolling your head or making jerky movements with your arms.

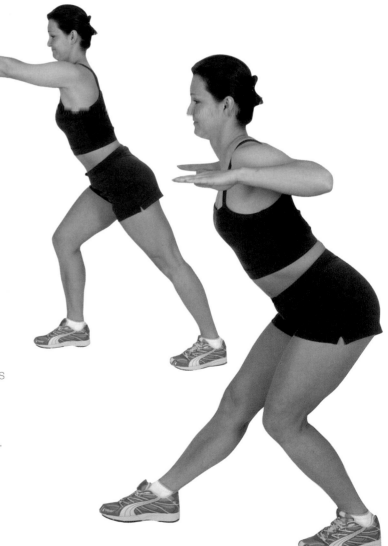

calves and arms

❶ Your aim in this movement is to stretch the calves, hamstrings, chest, and upper back.

❷ Start in a standing calf stretch (page 109), with both hands pointing out directly in front of you.

❸ Keeping your feet firmly on the floor, extend your elbows back and move into a standing hamstring stretch (page 119).

Perform this movement ten to twenty times on each leg, gradually increasing the range of movement.

lying trunk twists

❶ Lie on your back with both feet raised and in line with your hips, legs straight and feet together.

❷ Keeping your legs straight and in line with your hips, twist both feet from one side to the other, gradually increasing the movement, one twist every three seconds.

Aim for ten to twenty movements each side with your back fixed to the floor.

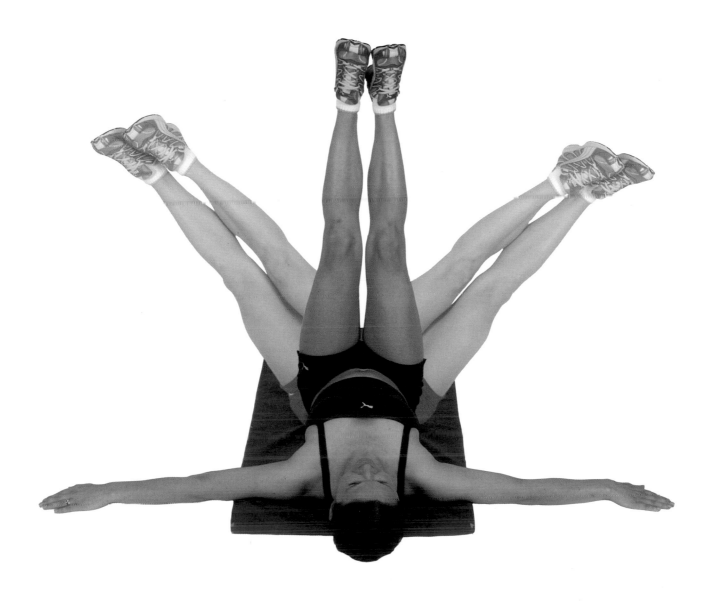

push-ups

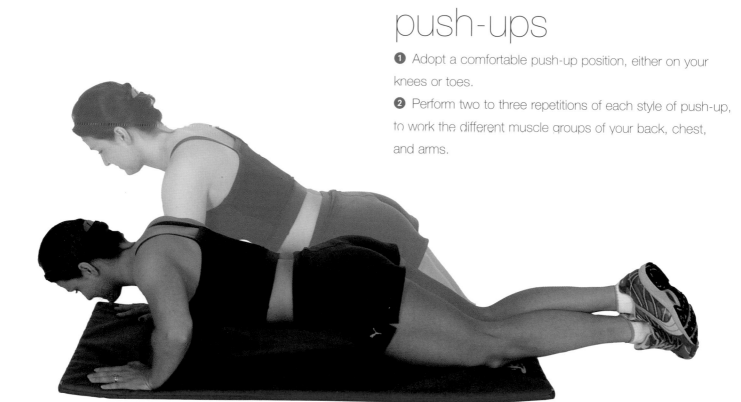

❶ Adopt a comfortable push-up position, either on your knees or toes.

❷ Perform two to three repetitions of each style of push-up, to work the different muscle groups of your back, chest, and arms.

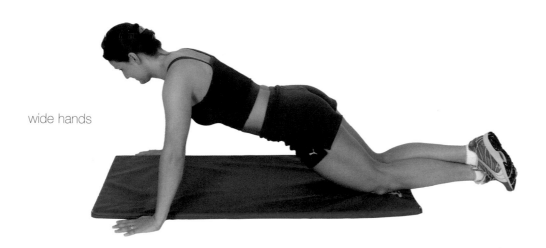

wide hands

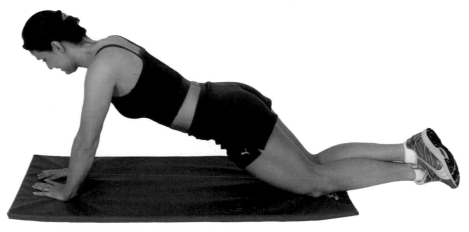

close hands, thumbs and index fingers forming a triangle

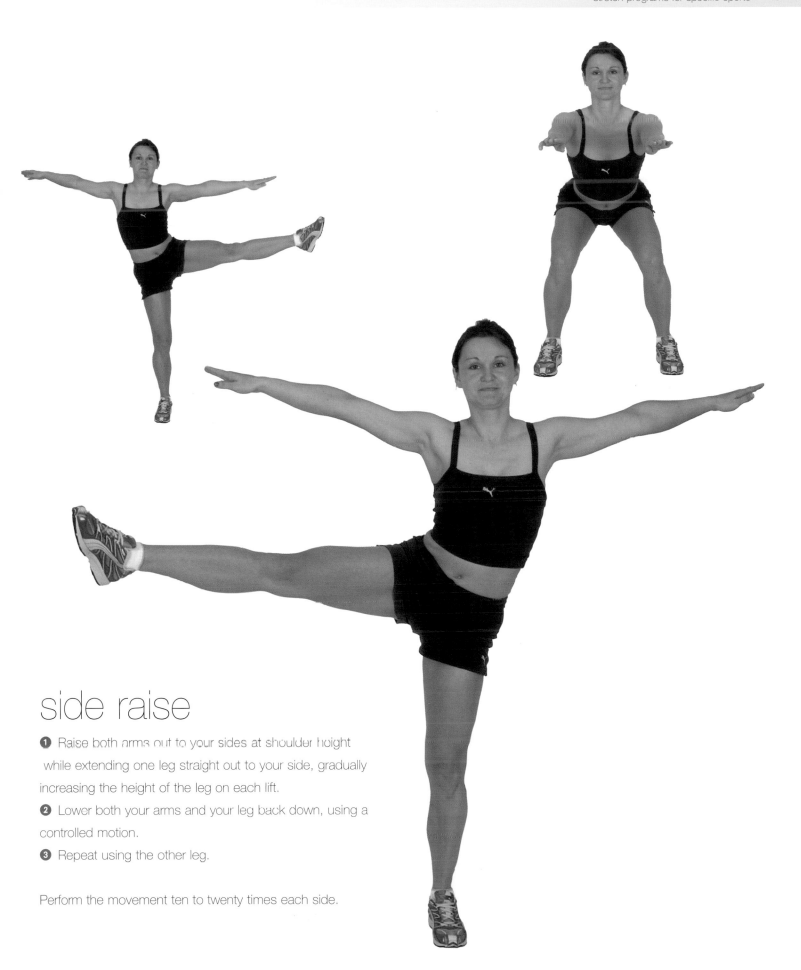

side raise

❶ Raise both arms out to your sides at shoulder height while extending one leg straight out to your side, gradually increasing the height of the leg on each lift.

❷ Lower both your arms and your leg back down, using a controlled motion.

❸ Repeat using the other leg.

Perform the movement ten to twenty times each side.

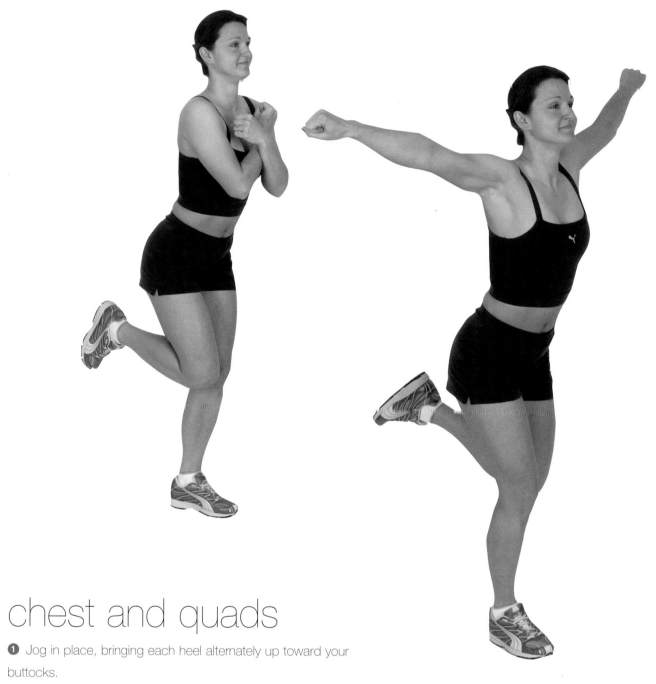

chest and quads

❶ Jog in place, bringing each heel alternately up toward your buttocks.

❷ As your heels come up, take your arms across your chest, and then out to the side, opening up your chest.

Perform this ten to twenty times on each leg, gradually increasing the range of movement.

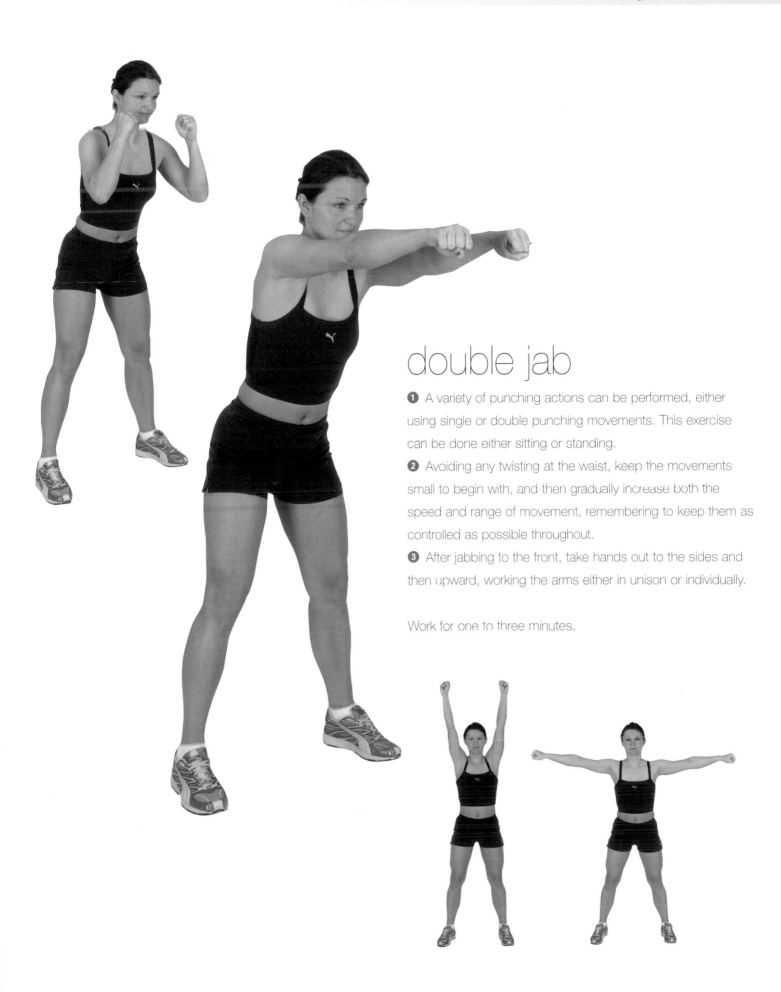

double jab

1 A variety of punching actions can be performed, either using single or double punching movements. This exercise can be done either sitting or standing.

2 Avoiding any twisting at the waist, keep the movements small to begin with, and then gradually increase both the speed and range of movement, remembering to keep them as controlled as possible throughout.

3 After jabbing to the front, take hands out to the sides and then upward, working the arms either in unison or individually.

Work for one to three minutes.

chest opener **diagonal arms**

❶ Stand with your feet shoulder width apart and your arms straight out to the side. Next raise one hand slightly higher than your head, and lower the other diagonally to the floor, until your hand is at hip level.

❷ Press both hands forward a few inches and then back, making sure you control the movement throughout and adjust the position of your hands—palms facing down, forward, or upward.

❸ Repeat this movement ten times on each side, then, still keeping the arms straight and the fingers pointed out, allow them to cross in front of you and then cross them behind you. This involves taking the high hand from head height to hip height, while taking the hip hand to head height.

❹ Breathe deeply through the motion, exhaling as you take your hands back in order to stretch your chest and bicep muscles.

Work this movement for one to three minutes.

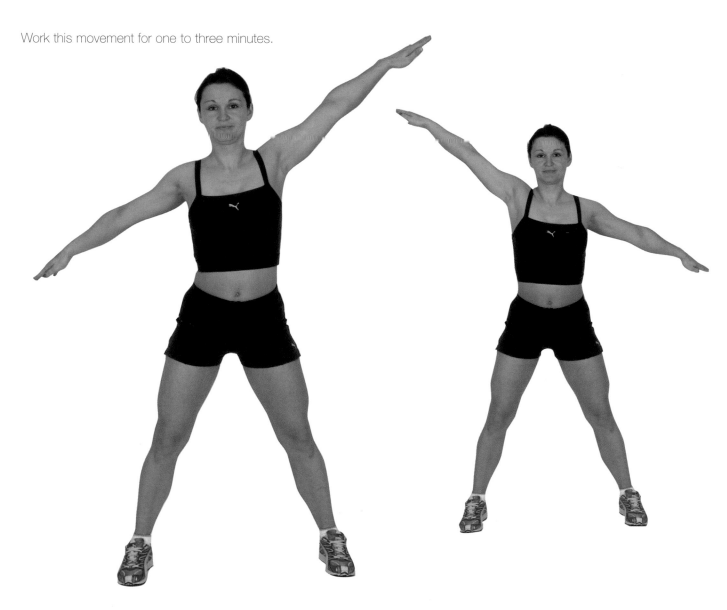

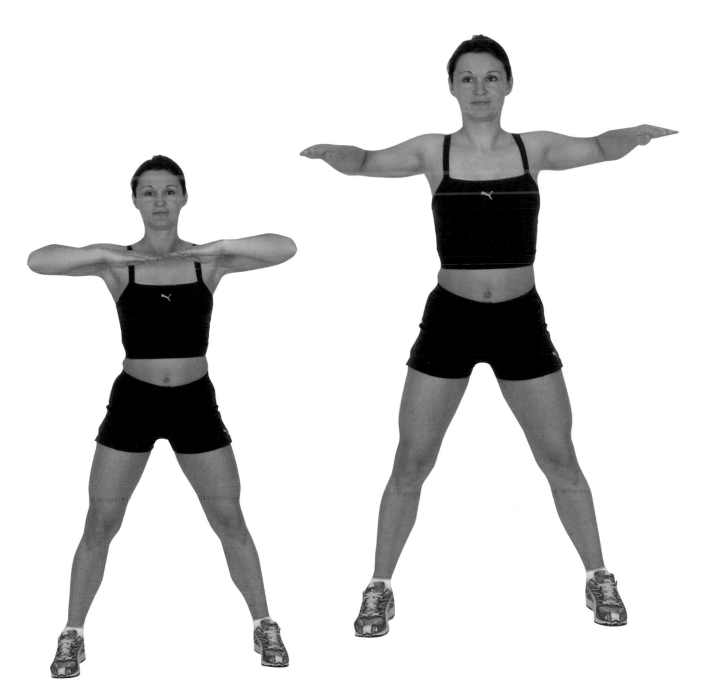

chest opener

❶ Stand with your feet pointing forward, double shoulder width apart, elbows at shoulder height, and your forearms parallel with the floor.

❷ Using smooth movements, extend the elbows back to the side of your body and then back behind you, keeping them straight and holding them at shoulder level. Concentrate on counting one second for each movement.

Perform ten to twenty repetitions, turning your palms inward and then outward to work different muscles of the chest.

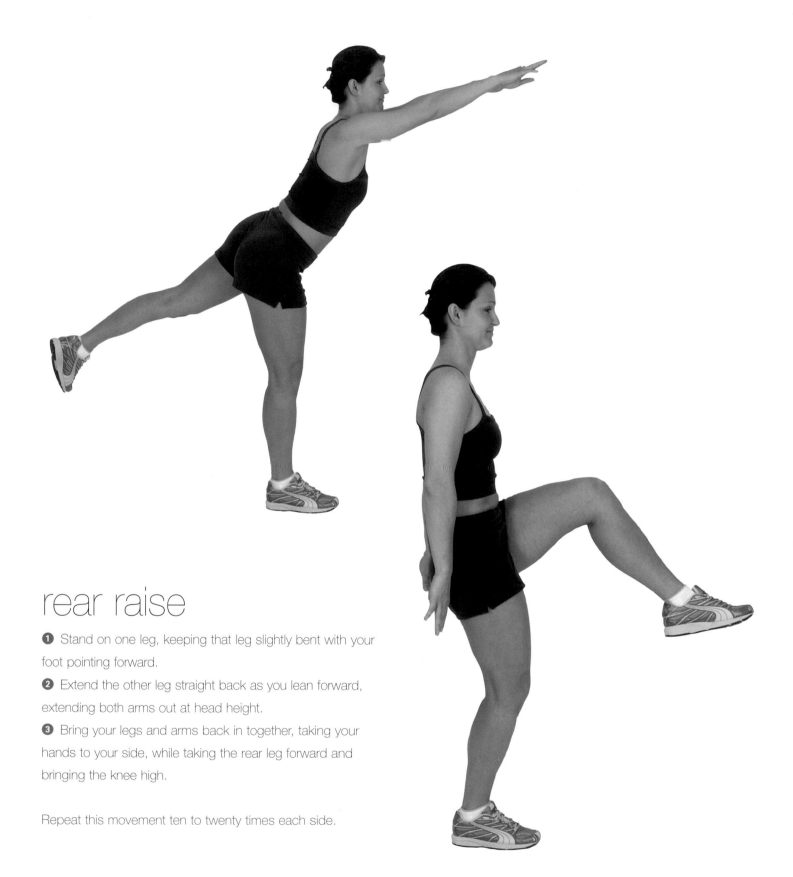

rear raise

❶ Stand on one leg, keeping that leg slightly bent with your foot pointing forward.

❷ Extend the other leg straight back as you lean forward, extending both arms out at head height.

❸ Bring your legs and arms back in together, taking your hands to your side, while taking the rear leg forward and bringing the knee high.

Repeat this movement ten to twenty times each side.

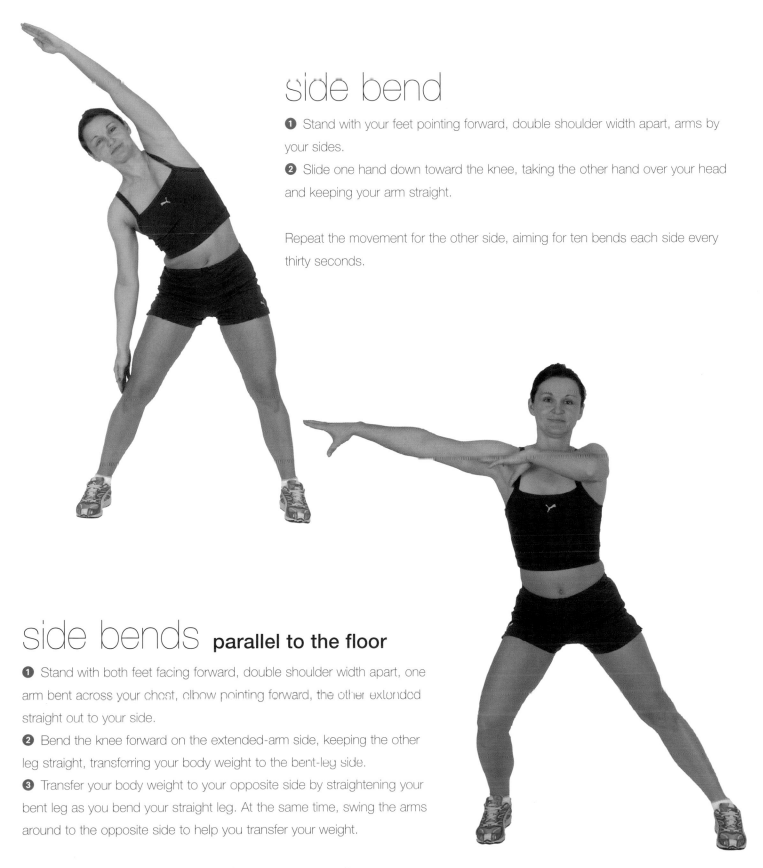

side bend

❶ Stand with your feet pointing forward, double shoulder width apart, arms by your sides.

❷ Slide one hand down toward the knee, taking the other hand over your head and keeping your arm straight.

Repeat the movement for the other side, aiming for ten bends each side every thirty seconds.

side bends **parallel to the floor**

❶ Stand with both feet facing forward, double shoulder width apart, one arm bent across your chest, elbow pointing forward, the other extended straight out to your side.

❷ Bend the knee forward on the extended-arm side, keeping the other leg straight, transferring your body weight to the bent-leg side.

❸ Transfer your body weight to your opposite side by straightening your bent leg as you bend your straight leg. At the same time, swing the arms around to the opposite side to help you transfer your weight.

Keep your back straight throughout this movement, repeating twenty to forty times in thirty to sixty seconds.

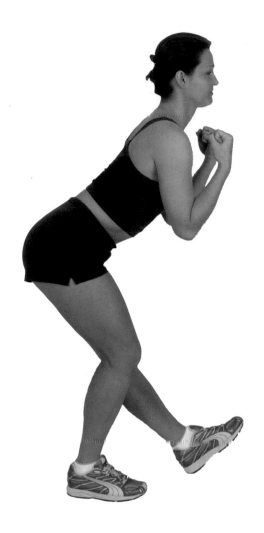

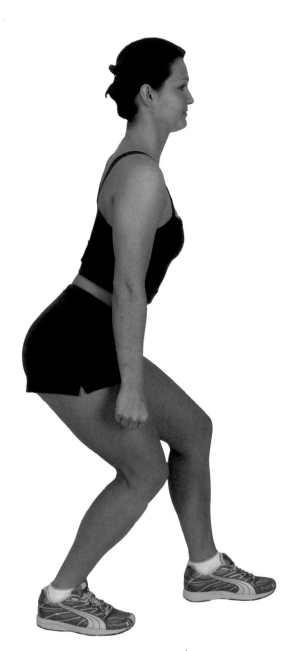

soleus and hamstring

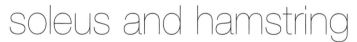

❶ Stand in the position for a normal hamstring stretch (page 119), with your front foot raised, both arms bent at the elbow, and your hands close to your shoulders.

❷ Lower your front foot and your arms while bending both legs in order to move into the soleus calf-stretch position (page 112).

Repeat the movement ten to twenty times each leg, at a rate of one bend every three seconds.

sprint

1 Working either on the spot or taking small steps forward, overexaggerate a sprinting action, raising one knee high off the floor, pointing the foot downward, and raising the opposite arm.

2 Keeping the other leg straight, come up on your toes, driving the raised arm up to head height, slightly forward of your body's centerline.

3 The fingers of both hands should be spread, with the remaining arm extended straight back behind you.

You can either work one leg at a time or use alternate legs, gradually building up both the speed and range for each action.

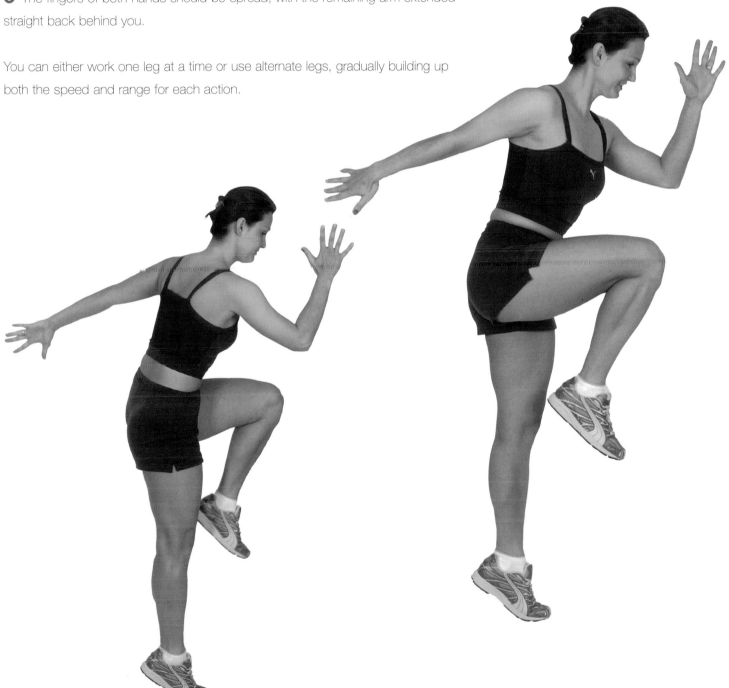

trunk rotation

❶ Stand with both feet double shoulder width apart, both feet facing forward, hands at shoulder height, one bent, with the elbow pointing forward, and the other out to your side. Turn your head to look along your arms.

❷ Rotate from your waist, keeping your back straight throughout and keeping your pelvis forward, while you gently swing the arms from side to side, alternating the extended arm as you do so.

Repeat twenty to forty times in thirty to sixty seconds.

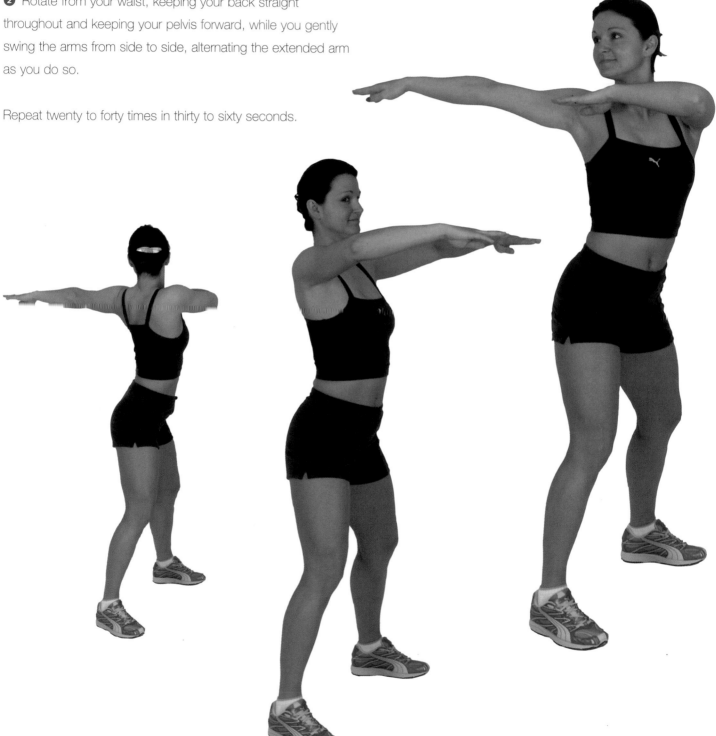

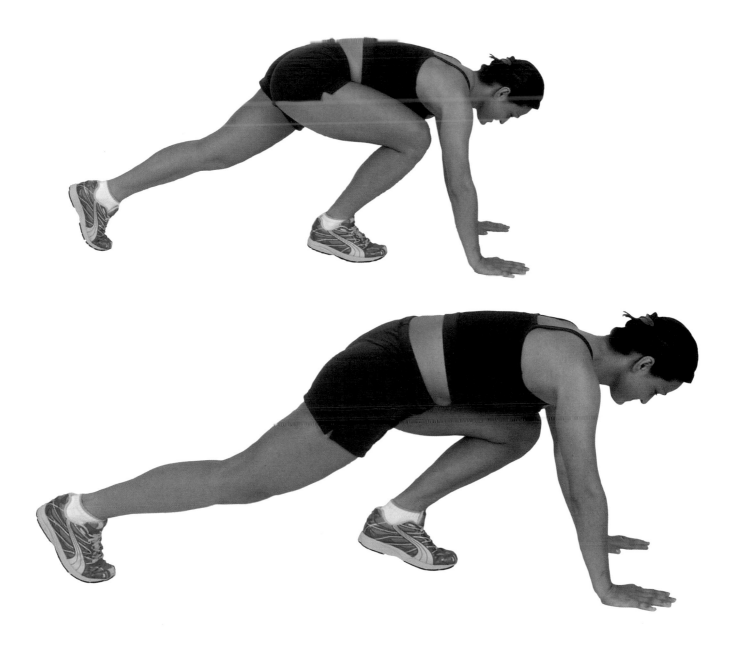

squat thrusts

❶ Place both hands flat on the floor, under your shoulder, with your fingers pointing forward.

❷ Staying on your toes, with your back parallel to the floor, extend one leg straight back, bringing the other up toward your chest.

❸ Alternate the legs, performing five to fifteen slow movements.

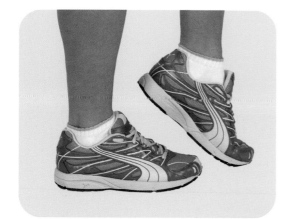

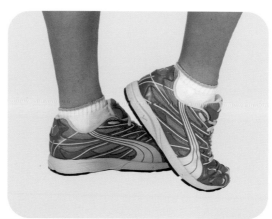

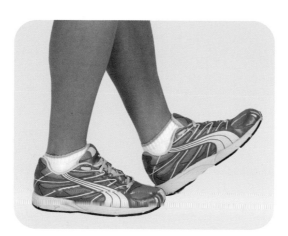

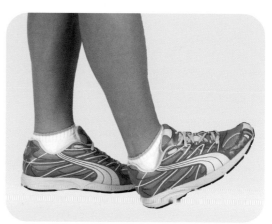

foot and heel raises

❶ Standing on the spot, lift each heel alternately off the floor, placing all your weight on your toes. Gradually increase the lift, holding the stretch for longer each time (try to hold it for two seconds).

❷ This action can be performed seated by applying pressure downward on your knees with your hands.

❸ Progress to a slow walk forward, taking small steps, placing your heel down first, and keeping your toes pointed upward for as long as possible.

❹ Contract your quadriceps as you point the toes upward. Take one step every three to five seconds, spending one to three minutes on each movement.

ladder drills

These drills are used to gain speed in footwork.

1 Lay out a rope ladder or chalk out an area with approximately fifteen-inch squares. Combining ladders so that you go both forward and sideways will give you rapid results. The numbers indicate the order to run in.

2 By performing these drills in both directions, you will soon realize that you are better on one side than the other. Work on your weaker side for greater improvement in your footwork.

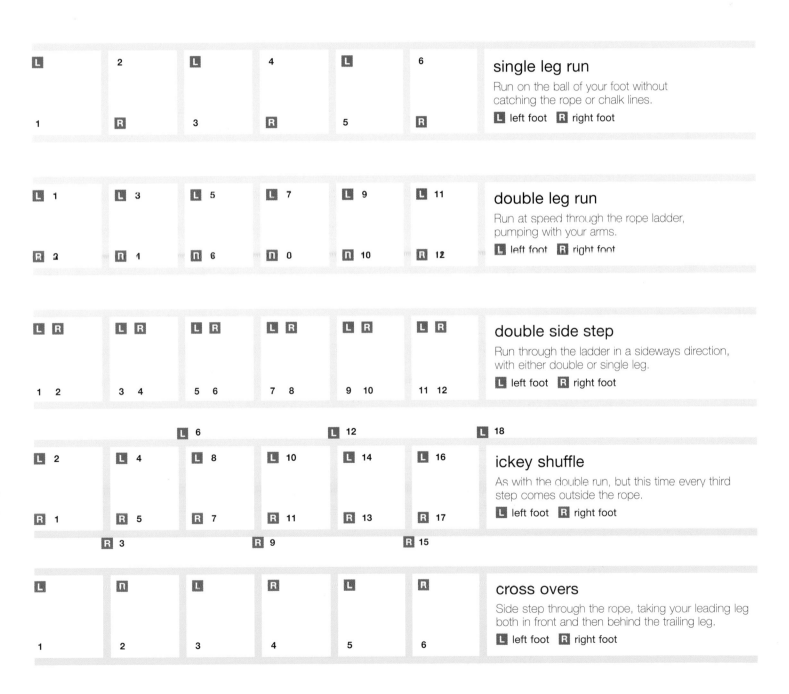

single leg run

Run on the ball of your foot without catching the rope or chalk lines.

L left foot **R** right foot

double leg run

Run at speed through the rope ladder, pumping with your arms.

L left foot **R** right foot

double side step

Run through the ladder in a sideways direction, with either double or single leg.

L left foot **R** right foot

ickey shuffle

As with the double run, but this time every third step comes outside the rope.

L left foot **R** right foot

cross overs

Side step through the rope, taking your leading leg both in front and then behind the trailing leg.

L left foot **R** right foot

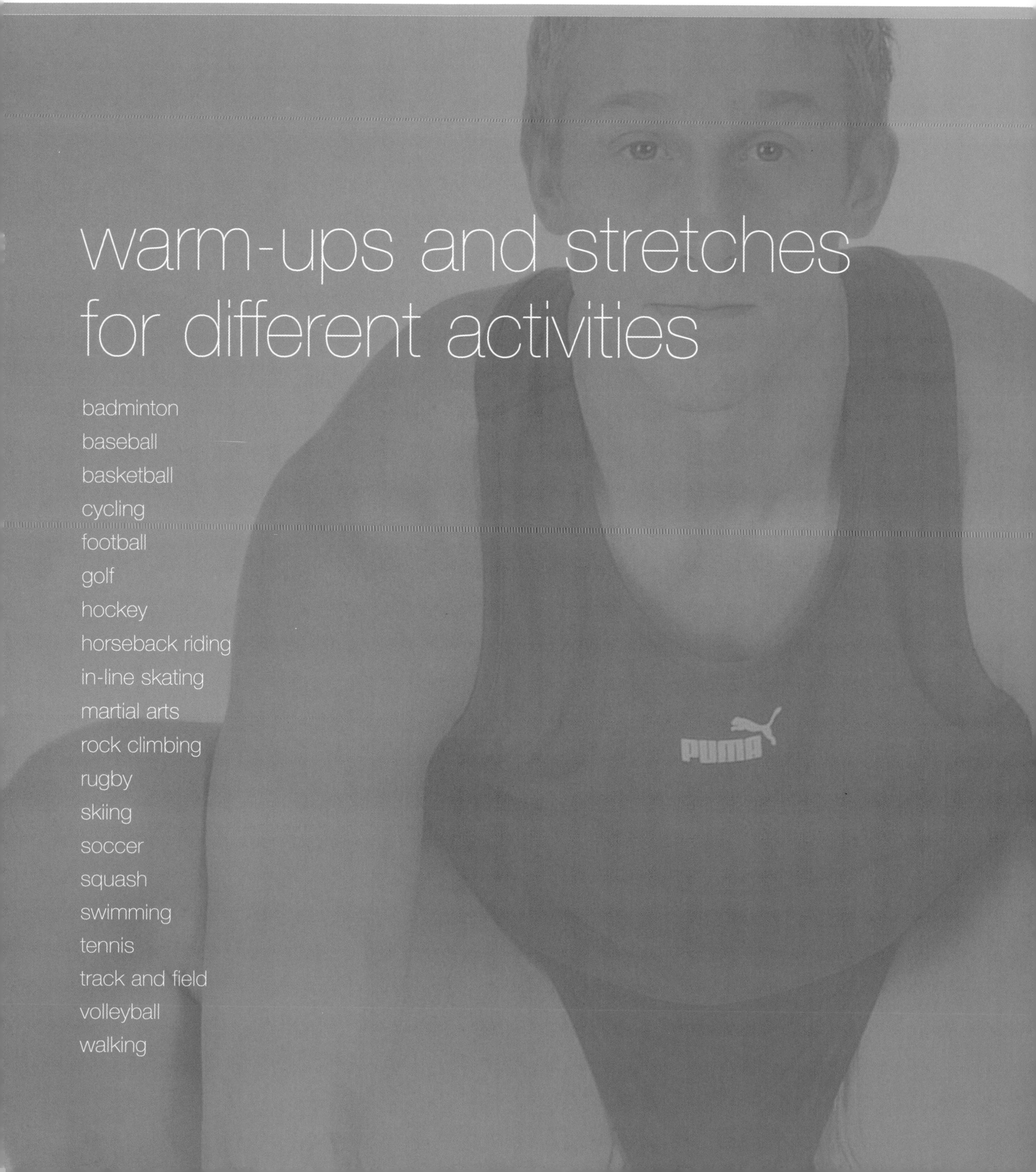

warm-ups and stretches
for different activities

badminton

baseball

basketball

cycling

football

golf

hockey

horseback riding

in-line skating

martial arts

rock climbing

rugby

skiing

soccer

squash

swimming

tennis

track and field

volleyball

walking

This section suggests a series of warm-up, stretching, and cool-down exercises that are appropriate for various activities.

warm-up

Perform this sequence of stretches only after you have warmed up the muscles; remember that your warm-up is the key to unlocking tight muscles, which are often the cause of injury.

start	soleus	normal stretch	quadriceps standing	side lunge	leg over
	page 113	page 119	page 101	page 93	page 82
	fetal position	spine curve	bar twist	cat stretch	elbows back
	page 36	page 44	page 43	page 35	page 77
	shoulder strangle	wall stretch	triceps	upward stretch	chin to chest
	page 67	page 62	page 63	page 68	page 52	finish

Hold each stretch for twenty to thirty seconds, breathing comfortably throughout.

cool-down

Once you have finished any form of physical activity, you should gradually allow your heart rate and breathing to lower to a comfortable level, where you can talk with ease. Light aerobic exercise, such as walking or easy indoor cycling is good.

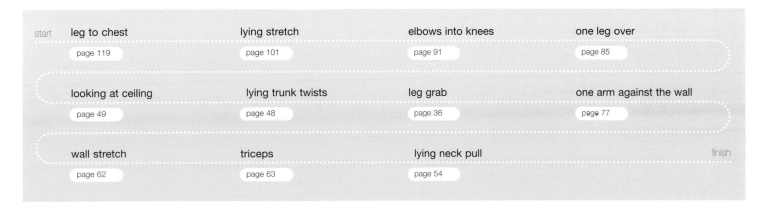

start	leg to chest	lying stretch	elbows into knees	one leg over
	page 119	page 101	page 91	page 85
	looking at ceiling	lying trunk twists	leg grab	one arm against the wall
	page 49	page 48	page 36	page 77
	wall stretch	triceps	lying neck pull	finish
	page 62	page 63	page 54	

Hold each stretch for a minimum of twenty to thirty seconds, breathing comfortably throughout. If specific areas are still tight, then repeat the stretch or look for other suitable stretches within the stretch menu.

badminton

Badminton is a sport with rapid actions and unmeasured aerobic activity. It involves approximately thirty to forty minutes of lunging, rapid forward and rear movements, high jumping, shuffling, striding, and uncontrolled landings, often at full extension with minimal rest periods. Common injuries include tennis elbow, achilles rupture, repetitive strain injuries to the wrist, and the highest level of eye injuries of all the racket sports, so always aim to wear some form of eye protection.

Avoid the warm-up method that is traditional to this particular sport, i.e, simply walking onto the court and hitting the shuttlecock a few times back and forth. Regardless of your level of ability, spend at least five minutes working on your mobility exercises, followed by a further ten minutes warming up, either by jogging lightly or, even better, jumping rope before beginning your static stretches on page 20.

Dynamic movements (see pages 130–149), using a controlled action, should follow the static stretching to help prepare you for the game. Depending on your level, you may also wish to perform the foot drills on page 149.

Prior to going onto the court, carry out some simple warm-ups. During periods of rest, keep moving, even between each point in the game—simply lifting and lowering the heel alternatively on each foot will help to relax the muscles of the leg, and thus reduce the risk of injury and allow for greater performance.

Use all the static stretches on page 20, and include the following to prepare you.

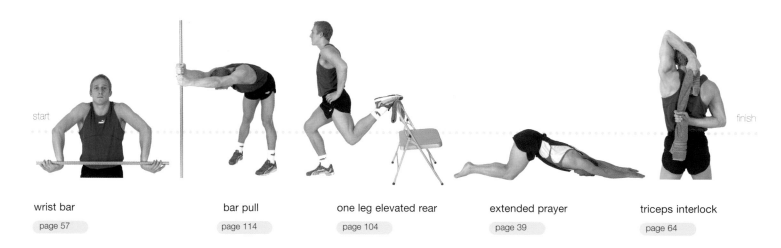

start   finish

wrist bar	bar pull	one leg elevated rear	extended prayer	triceps interlock
page 57	page 114	page 104	page 39	page 64

Always spend a minimum of five minutes cooling down—you could even try to finish the game five minutes early, and use the last five minutes to practice shots, allowing for your heart rate to come down gradually. Once again use the cool-down stretches on page 151, along with those suggested above to help prevent muscle soreness and injury. Aim to hold each stretch for fifteen seconds, then take a deep breath in and exhale, increasing the stretch for another fifteen seconds.

baseball

Baseball involves long periods of inactivity, whether you are fielding or batting. Active play consists of explosive power in the arm of the pitchers and fielders who are throwing the ball, while batting combines trunk and arm rotation with short bursts of sprinting. As you will be fielding and batting, perform movements appropriate to both in a fifteen-minute warm-up. Practice some light running and mobility exercises for the trunk, arm, and shoulders before performing the stretches on page 151.

To prepare for pitching, spend ten minutes skipping and performing swimming motions using the arms. Move on to simulate a throwing action, flicking the fingers out at the end of the movement, then progress to throwing a ball. Fielders should stretch and stay mobile while on the diamond—active dynamic stretching should continue throughout the game. The batting team is generally in a dugout so keeping the body warm can be hard. Wearing extra clothing will help. Perform dynamic stretching movements five minutes prior to walking out of the dugout. You will need to sprint between bases, so don't skip the stretches for your lower body.

fielders

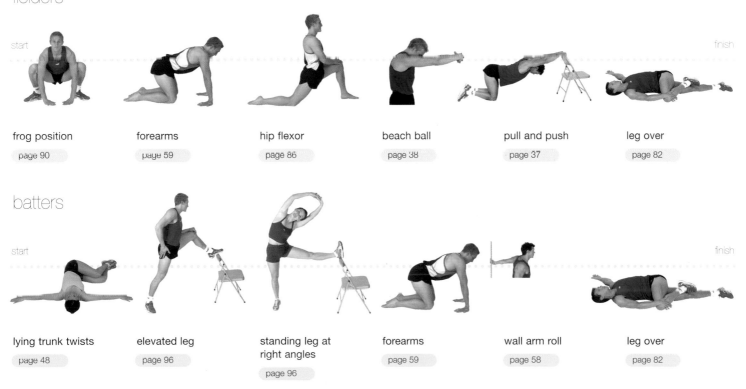

start   finish

| frog position | forearms | hip flexor | beach ball | pull and push | leg over |
| page 90 | page 59 | page 86 | page 38 | page 37 | page 82 |

batters

start   finish

| lying trunk twists | elevated leg | standing leg at right angles | forearms | wall arm roll | leg over |
| page 48 | page 96 | page 96 | page 59 | page 58 | page 82 |

Prior to stretching at the end of a game, players will require a gradual warm-up again, as the body will have been inactive. Jog lightly for five minutes before carrying out the cool-down stretches on page 151. Hold each stretch for fifteen seconds, take a deep breath in, and then exhale, increasing the stretch for another fifteen seconds.

basketball

Basketball is a sport that involves rapid, explosive movements that push the body to its limits in a combination of horizontal and vertical movements, often at high speed and with reduced body control. A well-structured flexibility and stretching program is essential, not only to reduce injury, but also to give a greater range of movement, increasing players' offensive and defensive capabilities. Correct footwear and clothing and a safe playing surface will all help reduce injury, the most common of which are sprains and strains to the ankles and knees, the lower back, hands, and wrists.

The warm-up phase should begin with five minutes of mobility exercises to lubricate all the joints before moving on to more active movements such as skipping, dribbling a ball, and light passing movements, for another ten minutes.

Stay warm throughout the stretching period and perform all the warm-up stretches on page 151, followed by the dynamic stretching movements on pages 130–149.

Time should then be spent on mind/body coordination and hand/eye drills. Practice your passing and shooting skills in order to make the central nervous system and your body's proprioception more effective from the start of your game.

Throughout a basketball game, players are often substituted and then brought back into the game at a moment's notice. So it's essential to stay actively warm and to continue to practice any shooting, passing, or ball handling drills. Sitting and watching the game will give your team support and allow you to watch your opposition's weaknesses, but you also risk rapidly cooling down and becoming less effective.

The cool-down and stretch period should be a gradual process to steadily reduce the heart rate. Wipe off any sweat and put on warm clothing before performing all the cool down stretches on page 151. Hold each stretch for fifteen seconds, then take a deep breath in and, on the out-breath, increase the stretch for another fifteen seconds.

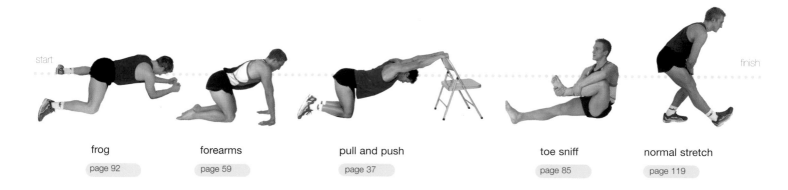

start | finish

| frog | forearms | pull and push | toe sniff | normal stretch |
| page 92 | page 59 | page 37 | page 85 | page 119 |

PNF stretching with a partner after the game, along with regular massage, is very helpful in maintaining the good range of movement that the game demands.

cycling

Cycling (either indoors on a stationary bike or outside in the open air) is an excellent form of exercise for the cardiovascular system (heart and lungs) and also provides a low-impact leg workout. Those cyclists who compete on the track or in short road races should spend five minutes warming up their joints with the mobility exercises on pages 16–19, and then a minimum of fifteen minutes actively warming up on a bike.

The bike warm-up should begin with a light gear, gradually increasing the cadence (pedal speed), and finally increasing the resistance.

Cyclists' injuries are often related to strains on the lower back, neck, and wrists, as these areas are often static throughout the ride. Try and avoid letting these muscles become sore by allowing them to have a simple stretch during your ride, for example, sitting upright for a few seconds or cycling out of the seat will help ease the tension.

After your warm-up phase, complete the following stretches prior to getting back onto your bike, and continue to stay warm while waiting for the start of the race. You should allow a minimum of thirty minutes to warm up and stretch if racing.

For cyclists who are simply going on a bike ride, spend time performing the mobility exercises, then, for the first five to ten minutes, cycle at an easy pace both in and out of the seat. At the earliest opportunity after this active warm-up, come off the bike in a safe place, (not in the road) and perform the following stretches.

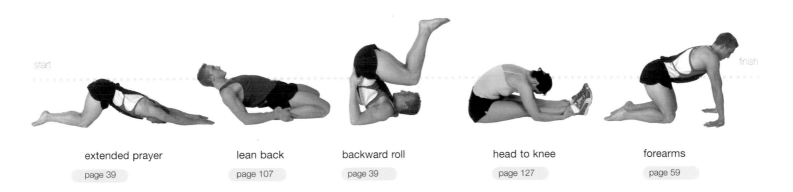

start   finish

| **extended prayer** | **lean back** | **backward roll** | **head to knee** | **forearms** |
| page 39 | page 107 | page 39 | page 127 | page 59 |

The cool-down period should consist of five minutes of light cycling, designed to bring the heart rate down, while sitting upright to ease any tension in the lower back.

On completion of your ride, wear warm clothing and carry out the mobility exercises for the back, shoulders, arms, and wrists again to help relax these areas. Carry out the static stretches on page 20, holding each stretch for a period of fifteen seconds before taking a deep breath and increasing the stretch as you exhale slowly.

PNF stretching on the back, hamstrings, and quadriceps (page 121), carried out once a week, will help prevent muscle shortening and thus give you greater flexibility, increased cycling ability, and reduce the chances of muscle soreness.

football

Football is unquestionably a contact sport. Sprains and strains are the most frequent injuries sustained among players, of which arms, hands, knees, and shoulders are the most common. All injuries should be treated at the earliest opportunity. Regular sports massage can help break down tissue that is scarred from heavy contact.

The nature of the game is such that players may spend long periods of inactivity on the bench before suddenly throwing their bodies at maximum effort into their opponents. The warm-up phase should be sufficient to warm and mobilize all joints and muscles prior to stretching, and players should continue to warm up throughout the game. Use the sidelines and spend at least two minutes in every ten jogging lightly, performing foot and hand drills with other players. Keep your body warm and hydrated while waiting to go onto the field and stretch whenever there is time to do so.

The stretches you perform after your warm-up should be static ones initially, followed by dynamic ones, to mimic the movements about to be performed.

start 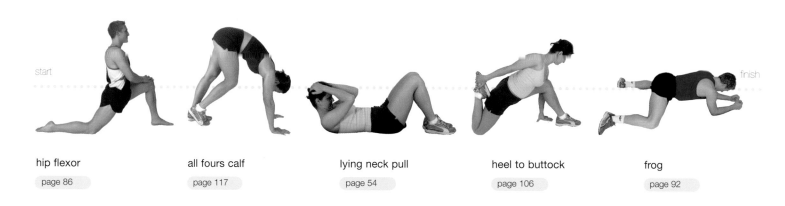 finish

| hip flexor | all fours calf | lying neck pull | heel to buttock | frog |
| page 86 | page 117 | page 54 | page 106 | page 92 |

Hold each stretch for twenty to thirty seconds, then, after every third stretch, spend thirty seconds running or skipping to keep the heart rate up, encouraging the body to stay warm.

Use the dynamic stretching routine and foot drills only after the static stretch. Prior to going onto the field, perform five push-ups and then ten alternate leg squat thrusts, at 100 percent effort.

Your cool-down should consist of drying any sweat away with a towel and putting on warm clothing to prevent a chill. Then perform the static stretches once more for thirty seconds, but this time relax the stretch after fifteen seconds, taking the stretch further. After every fourth stretch, walk around for thirty seconds, shaking the arms and legs (using a controlled action), to help keep blood from pooling that may result in dizziness. If possible perform the PNF stretches on page 121.

golf

Golfers at any level can reap the benefits that stretching can offer to their game. Played by all ages and by both men and women, the sport continues to grow in popularity.

Injuries in golfers tend to be due to overuse and poor technique. The leading side of the body (the side facing up the fairway) is more prone to injury, compared to the trailing side, because of the rotational and compression forces applied.

In comparison, professional golfers generally suffer overuse injuries to their hands and wrists, lower back, shoulders, and elbows.

Using appropriate equipment and wearing correct clothing (gloves and shoes) will help to minimize injuries associated with the sport.

Mobility work is a must for golfers—spend a minimum of ten minutes carrying out the exercises on pages 16–19, paying particular attention to the areas of the hands, wrists, arms, and trunk prior to beginning these dynamic stretches.

start   finish

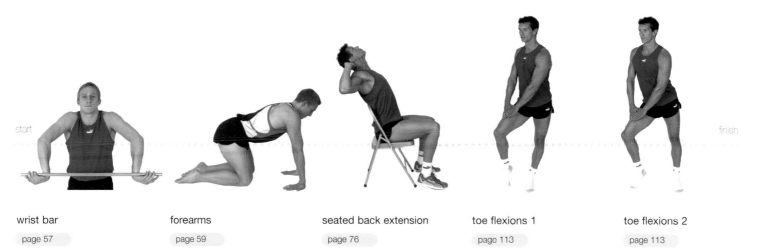

| wrist bar | forearms | seated back extension | toe flexions 1 | toe flexions 2 |
| page 57 | page 59 | page 76 | page 113 | page 113 |

Prior to playing a game, hit some balls on the driving range, gradually increasing the power you place into each shot.

With each shot off the green, take a few practice swings to maintain your body's flexibility, because, other than walking, the actual time spent in physical activity during a game of golf equates to less than a second per swing.

Prior to teeing off, perform the mobility exercises and dynamic stretches for the trunk, aiming to keep the wrists, shoulders, and elbows mobile throughout the game.

The cool-down phase should again consist of the mobility exercises for five minutes, followed by these stretches, which should be held for fifteen seconds before taking a deep breath to open up the lungs and then taking the stretch further while exhaling.

hockey

Correct footwear and protective clothing, shin guards, and a mouthguard will help reduce serious injuries. All players will reduce their injuries, and greatly improve their overall game, with a well-structured fitness program that includes stretching.

A minimum of thirty minutes should be allocated before a game or practice to your warm-up and stretching routine in order to reduce injury and increase physical performance for players.

The mobility exercises on pages 16–19 should be performed for a minimum of five minutes prior to going onto your aerobic warm-up. Begin with light skating around the rink without your hockey stick, gradually increasing the pace and implementing the following movements. Side steps facing in both directions, leaning forward while bringing your heels to your buttocks, raising your knees high, and running backward.

After ten minutes of active warm-up, begin the warm-up stretches on page 151, and then carry out the sports-specific stretches below. Stay actively warm by skating after every fourth stretch, this time with your hockey stick and puck, if you prefer.

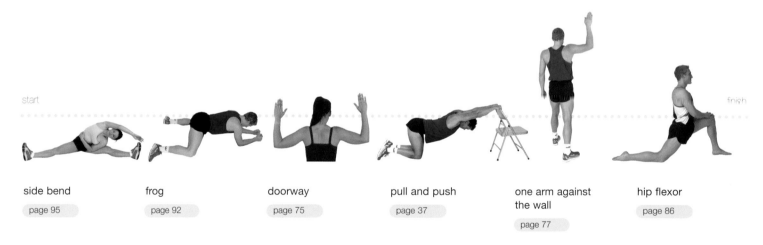

start   finish

side bend	frog	doorway	pull and push	one arm against the wall	hip flexor
page 95	page 92	page 75	page 37	page 77	page 86

Prior to going onto the rink, keep warm by wearing suitable clothing and performing the appropriate dynamic exercise. All substitutes should stay warm and stretch regularly throughout the game. During periods of rest (penalty box and intermissions), keep stretching in order to be at your maximum playing ability when the game recommences.

Your cool-down period should begin with five minutes of light skating wearing warm clothing to help lower the heart rate. Use the stretches on page 151, holding each stretch for fifteen seconds prior to inhaling and easing the stretch further as you exhale, holding for another fifteen seconds. The PNF stretches for the hamstring and lower back will help reduce muscle shortening in these areas, and as such should be performed after each session. Any injuries should be treated immediately, even before the cool-down, as frequently players may have sustained an injury, but the adrenaline of the game blocks out the pain.

horseback riding

Horseback riding injuries are often the result of a fall and commonly occur in the upper extremities, such as the wrist, elbow, and shoulder. Correct protective clothing for both the horse and rider is essential to reduce the risk of injury.

Those new to horseback riding will often feel sore in the inner thighs, upper quadriceps, and lower back, due to these muscles being worked continually in an isometric (static) mode in order to minimize movement while mounted on the horse. Isometric exercise places considerable strain on the muscles, and new or irregular riders should slowly increase the amount of time in the seat. Try riding for twenty minutes, then have a break to stretch out before riding for another twenty minutes.

Carry out the mobilization exercises (pages 16–19) prior to going into your warm-up phase. Your warm-up could involve the daily chores undertaken at most stables, i.e., mucking out, filling water buckets, and anything that will raise your heart rate slightly and enable the muscles to get warm through increased blood flow.

Once warm, do all of the stretches on page 151. Then use the following stretches prior to mounting and descending your horse to reduce muscle stiffness in prominent riding muscles. The warm-up should consist of gentle riding to allow the muscles to become accustomed to the movements for both horse and rider for five minutes.

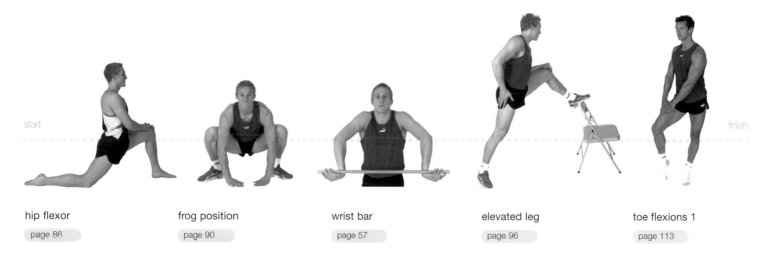

start   finish

| hip flexor | frog position | wrist bar | elevated leg | toe flexions 1 |
| page 86 | page 90 | page 57 | page 96 | page 113 |

Tired muscles become tight and lose flexibility, resulting in a poor riding position.

Your cool-down should consist of light riding for five minutes and then performing the mounting and descending stretches as soon as possible. After you have administered your horse, spend more time stretching out, repeating once again the descending stretches, followed by the cool-down stretches on page 151. Hold each stretch for fifteen seconds then inhale, gradually increasing the stretch as you slowly exhale.

in-line skating

Rapidly growing in popularity during recent years, in-line skating provides a good workout for your lower limbs, heart, and lungs, while placing little stress impact on your joints and muscles. Unfortunately many injuries do occur, mainly from falls or collisions. Simple procedures will minimize these injuries, however.

Having the correct size skates is essential for both balance and comfort. Avoid buying skates that place pressure on any part of your foot, as this pressure will increase when you skate. Before placing your skates on, dress yourself in protective clothing, knee and elbow pads, wrist guards, and a helmet.

Spend a minimum of five minutes going through the mobility exercises on pages 16–19, paying particular attention to the ankle and wrist joints.

Stretching with your skates on means your muscles are needed to aid balance—so they are unable to relax and stretch sufficiently. Recreational skaters should spend five minutes or more performing the dynamic movements on pages 130–149, after which they should do the following stretches.

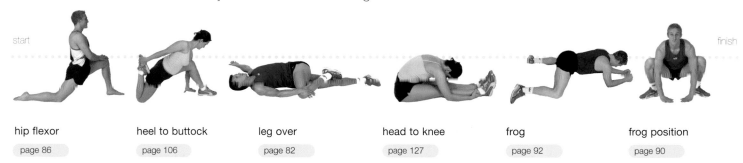

start .... finish

| hip flexor | heel to buttock | leg over | head to knee | frog | frog position |
| page 86 | page 106 | page 82 | page 127 | page 92 | page 90 |

Learning the basic skills such as how to stop and how to turn should be your first step.

Advanced skaters or speed skaters should perform a minimum of ten minutes light skating before removing their skates and performing the dynamic movements and stretches above.

Muscle strains tend to be in the inner thigh, buttocks, upper thigh, and lower back. Additional time stretching these areas both prior to and at the end of your skating session will prevent muscle soreness.

Begin skating with small movements, gradually progressing in order to allow the muscles worked to go through the movements in a controlled manner. The reverse should be done for your cool-down. Reduce your speed and also length of each movement to help lower the heart rate and prepare your body for the cool-down stretches on page 151. Hold each of these stretches for fifteen seconds, then take a deep breath and increase the stretch for another fifteen seconds. If you find that you are sore in particular areas, spend time stretching these muscles using the stretches available throughout this book.

martial arts

The movements in most martial arts are explosive and impact particularly on the legs. Continuous stretching of the complete body prevents many muscular injuries.

The nature of this sport, being one of self-defense and involving much physical contact, results in a high number of injuries from contact with your opponent, a weapon, or the floor. Protective clothing is essential and sparring should only take place between opponents of equal ability and under strict supervision.

With fitness playing a part in martial arts, training sessions should take the form of a high-energy, aerobic-style warm-up for twenty minutes. This should include running on the spot, skipping, push-ups, and squat thrusts to stimulate blood flow to the muscles.

Warm-up stretching is not suitable for most martial art movements, so look at performing the mobility exercises on pages 16–19 and then go on to the dynamic movements on pages 130–149. Once warm, begin each movement at a reduced intensity, gradually building up both the range of motion and velocity.

Perform the following stretches each morning or as cool-down stretches. Only begin after warming up. Breathe through the stretch, stretching a little further as muscles relax.

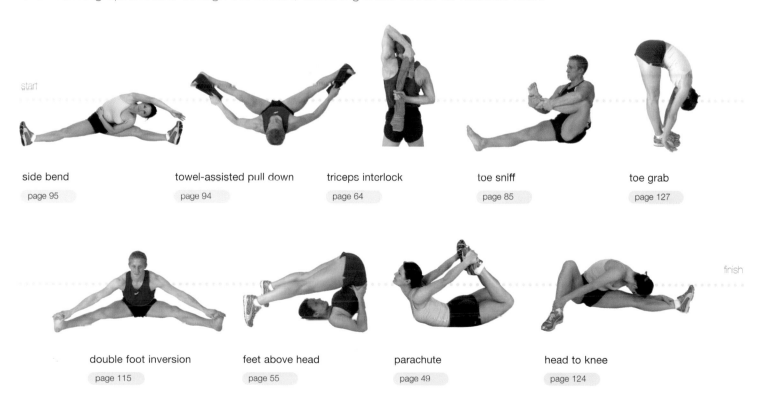

| side bend | towel-assisted pull down | triceps interlock | toe sniff | toe grab |
| page 95 | page 94 | page 64 | page 85 | page 127 |

| double foot inversion | feet above head | parachute | head to knee |
| page 115 | page 55 | page 49 | page 124 |

As you progress positively with your martial-arts training, you will naturally find yourself becoming more flexible, and as such you will need to increase the difficulty with new stretches specific to your martial art.

rock climbing

Rock climbing is demanding on the muscles of the wrists and forearms, which are often under tension throughout a climb, and on the back muscles, arms, and shoulders.

Stretching will enable you to perform difficult maneuvers that require a high degree of flexibility and good proprioception (body awareness). The joints and muscles in the forearms, wrists, and fingers suffer the most injuries, and time should be spent developing these areas physically and remedially.

The warm-up should consist of four phases. First, do the mobility exercises on pages 16–19, performing the movements for the fingers, wrists, and shoulders twice. Next, perform aerobic warm-ups to heat up your muscles. These can consist of walking to the start of the climb or a minimum of ten minutes of aerobic work, such as jogging in place. The stretching phase should enable you to take all your limbs to their full range of movement. As we all have a different flexibility, the key is to stretch, and climb within your limits, progressing safely and positively.

The final phase of the warm-up should include simple climbs to stimulate the muscles you are going to use and as such help return the blood back to the heart.

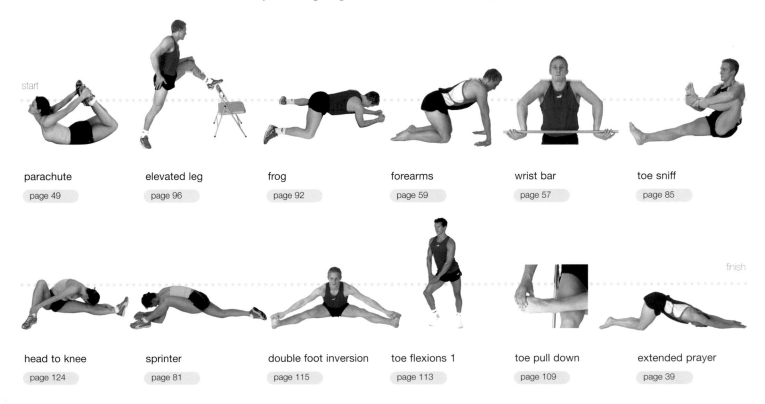

start

| parachute | elevated leg | frog | forearms | wrist bar | toe sniff |
| page 49 | page 96 | page 92 | page 59 | page 57 | page 85 |

finish

| head to knee | sprinter | double foot inversion | toe flexions 1 | toe pull down | extended prayer |
| page 124 | page 81 | page 115 | page 113 | page 109 | page 39 |

If you find that on these easy climbs your forearms feel "pumped" (full of blood) and ache, then spend more time warming up aerobically, followed by more stretching. The cool-down should begin with aerobic work to help circulate the blood, followed by your warm-up stretches, paying attention to your wrists, fingers, and forearms.

rugby

Rugby is one of the most physically demanding games in terms of potential player injuries. Tackling is where two-thirds of injuries occur, mostly to the lower limbs, especially the knee. Upper-body injuries such as dislocation and strains of the shoulder are also commonplace. It is essential to have a well-structured stretching program that also includes regular massage or physiotherapy to aid players in keeping fit and staying in shape before the game.

All training sessions should have a long warm-up and stretch, as every muscle will be used, normally beyond its natural limitations. Begin with the mobility exercises on pages 16–19. The aerobic warm-up should last at least fifteen minutes with simple ball-passing drills used to aid neuromuscular coordination while increasing blood flow to the muscles about to be stretched. Perform all of the stretches on page 151, and include the following in a static manner. After every fourth stretch, jog lightly for thirty seconds.

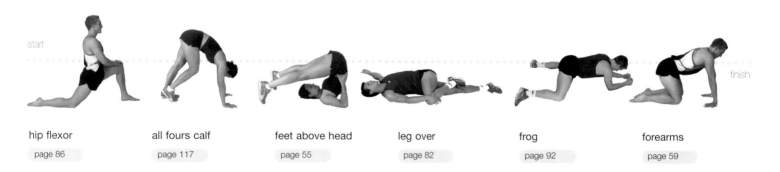

start

finish

| hip flexor | all fours calf | feet above head | leg over | frog | forearms |
| page 86 | page 117 | page 55 | page 82 | page 92 | page 59 |

After your static stretching, increase the heart rate again by performing the dynamic movements on pages 130–149, along with the foot drills on page 149.

It is wise for all players, including substitutes, to stay warm throughout the game, and also to drink suitable sports drinks to help their muscles perform correctly. All injuries, however trivial, should be treated at the earliest opportunity to help recovery.

As players are usually totally exhausted in the last ten minutes of play, the sound of the whistle tends to send everyone to the showers. Avoid the rapid drop in heart rate and blood flow around the muscles by spending just five minutes jogging lightly around the field to bring the heart rate down to a healthier level in which to stretch. Having a hot shower and removing restrictive protective clothing will aid in your postmatch stretch, using the cool-down stretches on page 151.

skiing

Time should be given prior to your vacation to concentrate on your fitness in order to get the full benefits from such a short period on the snow.

Beginners and less-experienced skiers have a higher risk of injury, with falls being the main cause. During a fall, aim to clench your fist away from the ski pole, to keep you from dislocating or damaging your thumb joint. Sprains, lacerations, fractures, and bruising are common types of injuries, with the knee, shoulder, and thumb being the main areas. Snowboarders have fewer knee injuries because of both feet being fixed onto the board, but they are vulnerable to head injuries so headgear is recommended.

Begin your warm-up with the mobility exercises on pages 16–19. You may feel particularly sore and stiff in certain areas of your body from the previous day's skiing, so spend extra time mobilizing these joints. Use an aerobic warm-up to help increase the blood flow in order to make the muscles more pliable. Follow this by the stretches on page 151 and also look at the ski-specific stretches below. Prior to skiing down each slope, do ten to fifteen standing squats. Start your skiing on easier runs, progressing gradually to warm up muscles and improve your coordination and balance.

Cool down fifteen minutes after your last ski run. You may wish to warm up aerobically, especially if your muscles are already feeling sore. Look at the stretches on page 151, holding each stretch for fifteen seconds before inhaling and extending the stretch for another fifteen seconds while you exhale.

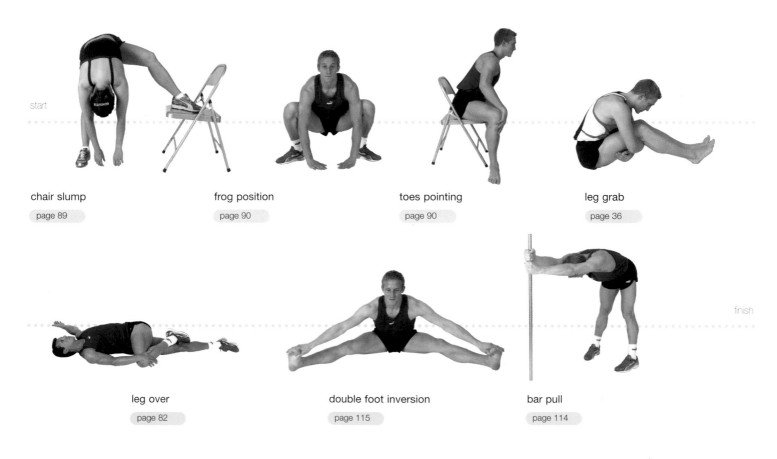

start

chair slump
page 89

frog position
page 90

toes pointing
page 90

leg grab
page 36

leg over
page 82

double foot inversion
page 115

bar pull
page 114

finish

soccer

The most common soccer injuries are to the knees, ankles, and feet, either as a result of a blow from another player or from the twisting movements placed upon these joints. Injuries can be acute (a single twist or blow) or due to overuse (a buildup of stress to a joint, muscle, or tendon). It is essential that protective clothing (boots with studs and shin guards) are worn. Those prone to ankle injuries should wear appropriate support. All players should spend a minimum of thirty minutes warming up and stretching, due to the vast array of movements and the explosive nature of the game.

The warm-up should begin with five minutes of mobility exercises, prior to light jogging. The pace should be slow, with warm clothing worn. After five minutes, change to sidestepping in both directions, leaning slightly forward, taking your heel toward your buttocks, finishing by jogging forward with a high knee lift and sprinting arm movement.

Static stretches should be carried out before the following stretches are performed.

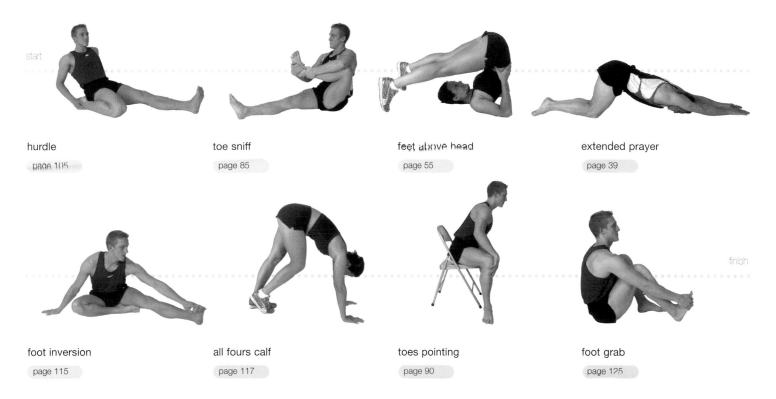

start

| hurdle | toe sniff | feet above head | extended prayer |
| page 105 | page 85 | page 55 | page 39 |

| foot inversion | all fours calf | toes pointing | foot grab |
| page 115 | page 117 | page 90 | page 125 |

finish

After an active warm-up and stretch, motor-neuron skills should be prepared by performing skill drills with a ball, passing it back and forth to the other players. Foot drills (see page 149), will prepare the body for movements associated with the game.

The cool-down should be a light jog around the playing field for five minutes before doing the cool-down stretches on page 151. PNF stretching, especially for the hamstrings and inner thigh muscles, should be carried out at least twice a week in the playing season, as these muscles are prone to becoming tight and injured.

squash

Squash is a popular racket sport that is very explosive in nature so players need to be quite fit. The nature of squash, with its sudden anaerobic periods, means that the risk of serious injury (cardiac-related) to unconditioned players is high. Regular players suffer from overuse injuries, especially to the wrist, forearm, and knee joints.

Start by doing mobility exercises on pages 10–19, followed by using a stationary bicycle for at least fifteen minutes. Alternatively, try skipping or light jogging.

Use the stretches on page 151, then perform the following squash-specific stretches.

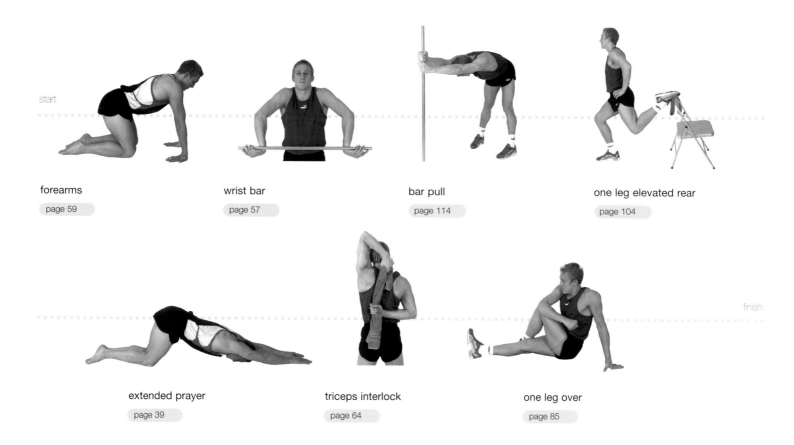

start

forearms

page 59

wrist bar

page 57

bar pull

page 114

one leg elevated rear

page 104

finish

extended prayer

page 39

triceps interlock

page 64

one leg over

page 85

Prior to walking onto the court for the general five-minute warm-up, perform some dynamic movements and foot drills (page 149).

Squash is often played in team matches. Once your match has finished, work on your cool-down to avoid sore muscles and the risk of blood pooling, which causes dizziness. Spend five minutes bringing your heart rate back to normal levels by walking or light cycling prior to performing the cool-down stretches. If you're in a second match, hold each stretch for fifteen seconds, and stay warm, taking in fluid before warming up and stretching again for fifteen minutes prior to your second match. Once you have finished playing, perform the cool-down stretches, holding each for fifteen seconds before inhaling and extending the stretch for another fifteen seconds as you exhale.

swimming

Swimming is an excellent all-around aerobic and muscle conditioning sport, especially suited for rehabilitation due to the buoyancy given by the water.

Injuries associated with swimming are due to overuse and poor technique, with the shoulder area being the most prone to serious soft tissue or muscular injury. Breaststroke can cause injury to the medial ligament of the knee due to the whipping action. Minimizing breaststroke distance by cross-training with other strokes, ensuring adequate warm-up, and increasing training distance gradually will reduce the risk of such injury.

Competitive swimmers will tend to swim year-round, often twice a day for up to two hours a session. Look for signs of overtraining, such as poor sleeping habits, increased resting heart rate, fatigue, muscle soreness, and lack of motivation.

A well-structured stretching program should become an essential part of any serious swimmer's training routine. As with all stretching, the muscles will need to be warmed, ideally with a combination of passive (warm shower) and active (aerobic) warm-up.

Most competition pools will have a training pool, which will enable swimmers to warm up actively prior to racing. During training sessions, warm-up swimming drills should always be included, such as 4 x 100-yard swims with all strokes, followed by leg kicks and hand drills. Likewise at the end of your session, time should be spent cooling down and relaxing the muscles with controlled slower swim strokes.

Noncompetitive swimmers will benefit from spending five minutes performing the mobility exercises on pages 16–19, and then a minimum of five minutes doing the dynamic movements on pages 130–149.

The following stretches should be performed both before and after each session, holding each stretch for fifteen seconds, then taking a deep breath and repeating for another fifteen seconds while increasing the stretch.

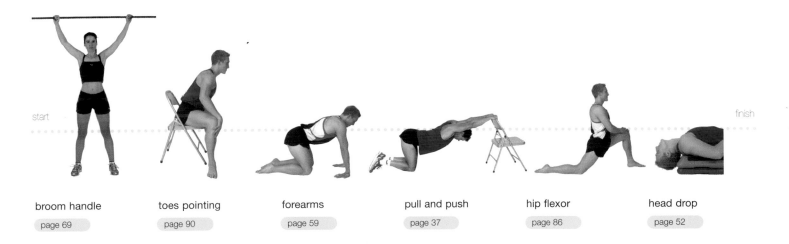

start ... finish

broom handle — page 69

toes pointing — page 90

forearms — page 59

pull and push — page 37

hip flexor — page 86

head drop — page 52

tennis

Tennis requires quick acceleration, twisting, rapid breaking, explosive arm actions and pivoting, putting the whole body under stress. Modern equipment has helped reduce injuries, with larger, lighter, stiffer rackets that are able to absorb the impact forces, and as such reduce the vibrations that will travel into the wrist. Correct grip size for your racket is essential to reduce the risk of injury.

Begin your warm-up routine with the mobility exercises on pages 16–19. Next, warm up aerobically for at least ten minutes by either skipping, light jogging, or cycling.

Stay warm while using the warm-up stretches and these sport-specific stretches.

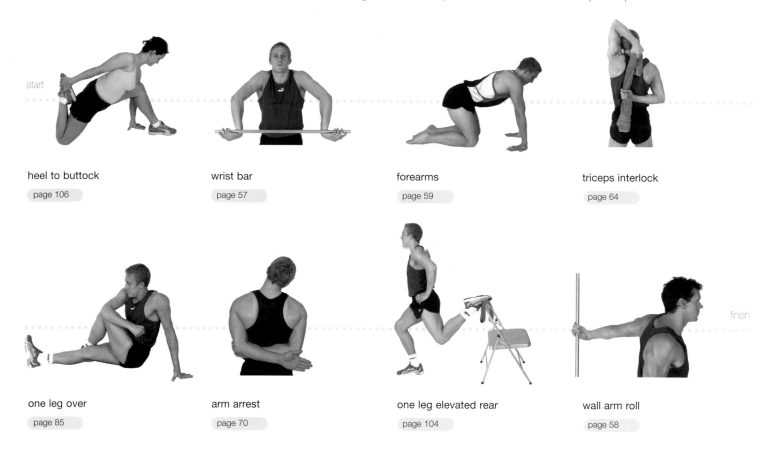

start

heel to buttock

page 106

wrist bar

page 57

forearms

page 59

triceps interlock

page 64

one leg over

page 85

arm arrest

page 70

one leg elevated rear

page 104

wall arm roll

page 58

finish

After every sixth stretch, spend thirty to sixty seconds jogging lightly to enable the muscles to stay warm and pliable. Once you have completed all of the static stretches look at the dynamic stretches on pages 130–149, and spend five minutes doing these.

Begin playing your practice shots to help your hand/eye coordination and neuromuscular system. Begin your play with easy shots from the baseline before practicing net shots. Once you've warmed your serving arm, work into your serve.

Commence your cool-down as soon as you finish, with five minutes of light jogging to circulate the blood in the lower legs, and to reduce the heart rate gradually. Finally, perform the cool-down stretches on page 151.

track and field

The different disciplines associated with track and field have the same causes for injury.

• Poor technique. Whatever level you compete at, improvements can always be made in your technique. Having a qualified, experienced coach to give you advice is invaluable in helping to prevent injuries and increase your performance.

• Overtraining or exertion. Vary your training sessions to avoid training sore muscles. Understand your limitations and fitness level and increase your performance gradually.

• Inappropriate clothing. Wear the correct clothing for your event. A range of footwear and protective clothing is available, designed to increase performance and avoid injury.

• Weather and track conditions. Keep yourself and any performing surface and equipment dry. During cold conditions, your muscles will take longer to warm up, so spend sufficient time warming up correctly, and once warm, stay warm with appropriate clothing and continual stretching/exercise, especially during throwing/jumping events. Remain hydrated with suitable sports drinks or water.

high jump and pole vault

Requiring high levels of flexibility and technically very demanding, both of these events should be coached and supervised. Implementing regular stretching and mobility exercises can reduce injuries from muscular strain, especially in the lower back.

Begin your warm-up with the mobility exercises on pages 16–19, prior to light jogging to circulate blood flow, minimum ten minutes, followed by warm-up stretches.

Perform the dynamic movements on pages 130–149. High jumpers should aim to carry out vertical knee lifts, gradually increasing height from their jumping leg, while vaulters should be making suitable adjustments to both run-ups and pole suitability by practicing at a reduced intensity on the pole vault runway.

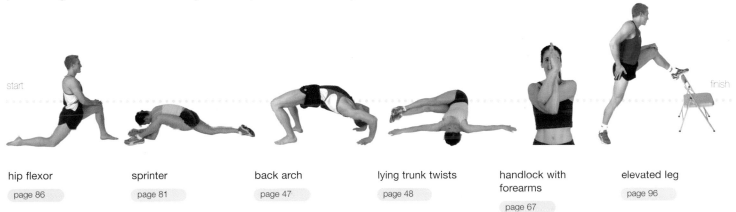

start   finish

| hip flexor | sprinter | back arch | lying trunk twists | handlock with forearms | elevated leg |
| page 86 | page 81 | page 47 | page 48 | page 67 | page 96 |

Cool down with a light jog for five minutes to revitalize the muscles and increase blood flow prior to performing the cool-down stretches on page 151.

running 800 meters up

Lower leg injuries are commonplace from overtraining (shin splints). The stresses placed on the body are different as the race distance increases, with aerobic and anaerobic fitness levels being important, especially in the later stages of a race.

Sufficient time should be spent preparing for your run to enable you to race at an optimum level. Light jogging for at least fifteen to twenty minutes should be carried out after the mobility exercises on pages 16–19, followed by the warm-up stretches on page 151.

Keep your muscles warm by continually jogging lightly, performing the dynamic movements on pages 130–149.

Cool down with light jogging for ten minutes, followed by the cool down stretches on page 151. Use different stretches from the book to alleviate any tension.

sprinting and hurdles

Due to the explosive nature of this sport, muscular strains are commonplace in sprinting and hurdling events, which is why it is essential to spend sufficient time warming all the muscle groups. Keep them both passively and actively warm throughout what can be a long day, especially if competing in numerous sprint heats, finals, and relays.

Begin your warm-up with light jogging, wearing warm clothing to help increase body temperature for at least ten minutes. Perform all the mobility exercises on pages 16–19 and the warm-up stretches on page 151 prior to the dynamic movements on pages 130–49. Perform these sprint/hurdle specific stretches both before and after you run.

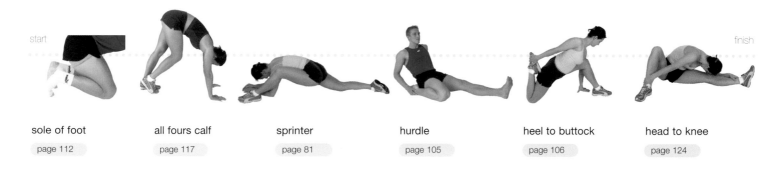

start					finish
sole of foot	all fours calf	sprinter	hurdle	heel to buttock	head to knee
page 112	page 117	page 81	page 105	page 106	page 124

Once fully warm, practice your running technique, focusing on your movements (knee lift/stride length) rather than speed, then practice your starts at a reduced intensity, gradually increasing your power efforts in order to be fully prepared both physically and mentally at least five minutes prior to your race.

Begin your cool down immediately after your race, wearing suitable clothing to keep the muscles warm and supple, then carry out the cool-down stretches on page 151.

throwing

Explosive power in the arm and shoulder muscles combined with rapid twisting from the hips and forceful breaking in your front leg places tremendous strain on the muscles and joints, especially in the throwing arm, opposite obliques, and lower back. Suitable supports are now specially designed for throwing events; however, make sure that these fit well and are used in training sessions prior to competition, as they can be restrictive.

Your warm-up needs to work all muscle groups, particularly the throwing shoulder. Skipping, rowing on an indoor rowing machine, or light jogging with imitation arm swimming movements should be performed for a minimum of ten minutes after the mobility exercises on pages 16–19.

Use the warm-up stretches on page 151, then continue with the dynamic movements, concentrating on areas that you use during your specific throwing event. Perform the following throwing stretches prior to simulating your throws at a reduced intensity.

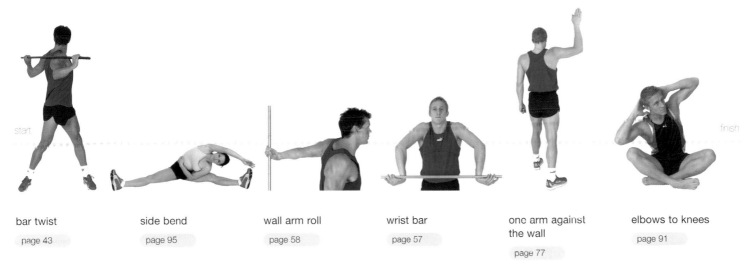

start   finish

| bar twist | side bend | wall arm roll | wrist bar | one arm against the wall | elbows to knees |
| page 43 | page 95 | page 58 | page 57 | page 77 | page 91 |

Stay warm and mobile throughout, continuing to stretch and take in both fluid and light sports snacks in order to keep blood sugar levels high and muscles supple and relaxed.

Cool down with five minutes of light rowing, skipping, or jogging with swimming movements prior to performing the cool-down stretches on page 151.

All athletes will benefit from implementing an extra stretching session into their weekly routines, especially during the competition period at both the beginning and end of the season.

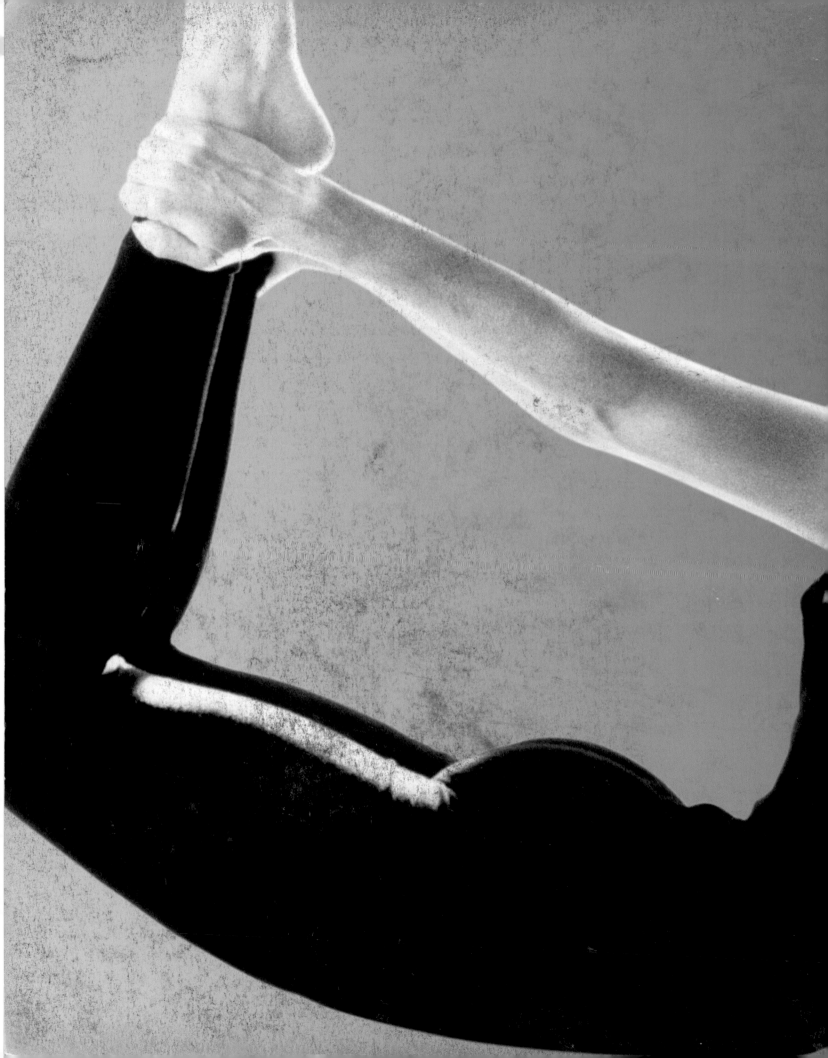

stretch routines
for everyday life

quick stretches

These combination stretches should be the absolute minimum prior to taking part in any form of physical activity.

As with all stretching, they are best performed once the muscles have been given a chance to warm up, ideally five minutes into the exercise. If time is really a problem, then work gradually into your workout or physical activity, ensuring you allow the four minutes it takes to carry out these quick combination stretches.

Hold each stretch for fifteen seconds, breathing comfortably throughout, then take a deep breath and increase the stretch a little further. A full description on how each stretch should be performed is given on each stretch's relevant page.

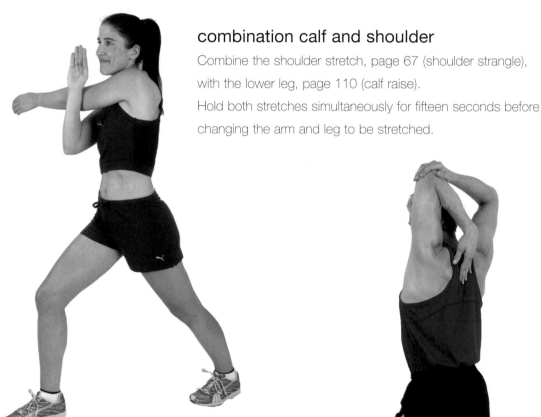

combination calf and shoulder

Combine the shoulder stretch, page 67 (shoulder strangle), with the lower leg, page 110 (calf raise).

Hold both stretches simultaneously for fifteen seconds before changing the arm and leg to be stretched.

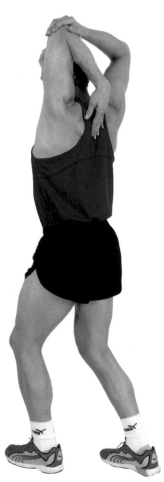

combination soleus and triceps

Combine lower leg soleus, page 112, with triceps, page 63. Hold each stretch for fifteen seconds, then repeat on the other side.

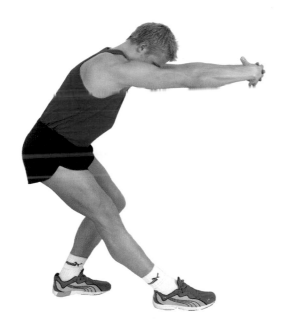

combination hamstring and back

Combine normal stretch, page 119, with beach ball, page 38.
Hold the stretch for ten to fifteen seconds, then repeat with
the same leg, this time raising your front toes up, while
swapping the inner and outer hands over.

combination hamstring and chest

Perform with the opposite leg as used above, with
the elbows back stretch, page 77.
Hold the stretch for ten to fifteen seconds, before
relaxing and then repeating, this time taking the
elbows closer together, and your foot raised.

combination neck and quads

Perform the quadriceps lying face down on page
101. While stretching the quadriceps, slowly
apply a steady pressure on the side of your head
in order to stretch the neck.
Hold the stretch for ten to fifteen seconds, then
repeat on the other leg and neck muscles.

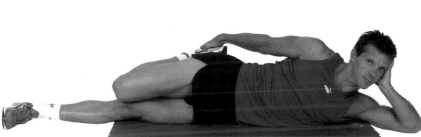

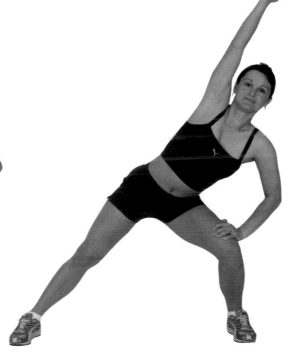

adductors and obliques

Combine the side lunge, page 93, with a stretch to your
shoulders and obliques by extending one arm up straight
above your head.
Hold the stretch for fifteen to twenty seconds, then repeat on
the other side.

back care

Lower back pain is the second most frequent cause of lost work days in adults, with four out of five adults experiencing problems at some point in their lives.

It is often caused by excessive strain due to poor posture, being overweight, or lifting incorrectly. For some, especially the elderly, enduring back pain may be due to arthritis or loss of bone density (osteoporosis), muscular strength, and flexibility.

Regular exercise, especially swimming if you suffer from back pain, will help keep your muscle mass and bone density from decreasing.

Use the correct lifting technique and get help if the object is awkward. Always remember to keep your back straight, lifting with your larger leg muscles.

Maintain a good posture, regardless of whether you are standing or sitting. Avoid staying still and keep the back mobile. While sleeping, go for a firm mattress that enables your spine to remain straight, not sinking into the bed.

Persistent backaches are often a result of obesity, which can place undue strain on the spine, and emotional stress, which causes individuals to unconsciously tense their muscles.

Strengthening and stretching the muscles of the lower back and abdominal area will help keep back pain from occurring. Lower back pain can be uncomfortable, but is not life-threatening. If this pain is associated with leg weakness or numbness, or bladder or bowel problems, there may be pressure on your nervous system. Seek medical advice

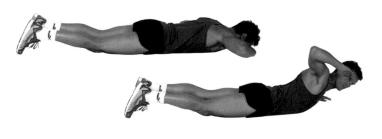

one arm dorsal raise

• Lie on your front, keeping your toes on the ground and placing one hand and forearm flat on the floor with the other hand resting on your forehead, palm facing the floor.

• Slowly lift one shoulder off the floor with your elbow pointing upward, keeping the other forearm flat on the ground.

• Lower under control and repeat five to fifteen times each side, one repetition every two seconds.

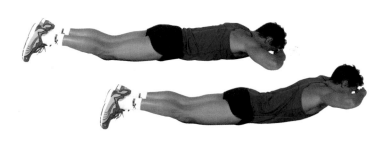

dorsal raise

Progress to performing two arm dorsal raises; remember to keep both feet in contact with the floor at all times.

simple dorsals

• Cross one foot over the other leg, resting it upon the thigh.

• Extend the arm of the crossed-leg side outward; palm facing down to the floor.

• Support the weight of your head with your other hand, keeping your chin off your chest and avoiding pulling on your neck.

• Slowly take your supporting elbow up toward your opposite knee. Avoid forcing the movement and travel as far as your abdominal strength allows. Repeat five to fifteen times each side.

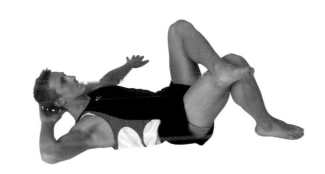

simple sit-ups

• Bend your legs to ninety degrees, resting your feet either on the floor or across a raised platform.

• Support the weight of your head with both hands, keeping your chin off your chest.

• Begin the exercise by lifting your shoulders off the floor, keeping your elbows out to your sides and lifting your head only six to twelve inches off the floor.

• Perform ten to twenty repetitions, one every two seconds.

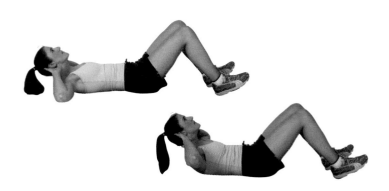

hand through

• Rest both knees on the floor, under your buttocks, while keeping a straight back. Support your upper body by placing one hand on the floor.

• Extend the other arm across your body, twisting slowly at your waist to take the hand out to your opposite side. Repeat five to ten times each side.

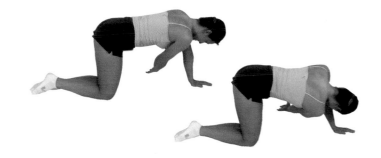

pluto sniffs

• Rest on all fours, keeping your knees shoulder width apart, and your hands under your shoulders.

• Keeping your knees and hands in contact with the floor, twist from your sides, looking over one shoulder toward your hip.

• Alternate from one side to the other in slow steady movements, gradually increasing the range of movement.

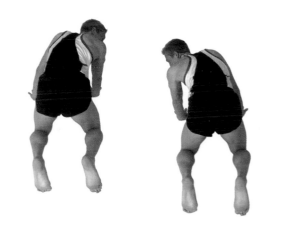

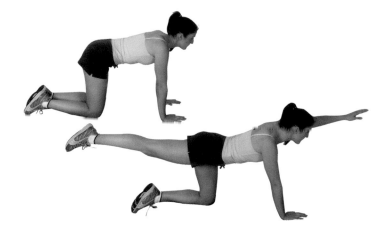

superman

- Rest on one knee and the opposite hand, keeping the knee below your hip and hand below your shoulder.
- Extend your other arm straight out to your front, while extending the opposite leg to your rear.
- Bring both your arm and leg back inward and repeat either on the same side or alternate sides, performing ten to twenty repetitions each side.

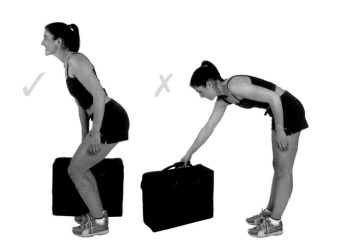

correct lifting

- Lift using your legs to initiate the movement, rather than your lower back.
- Stand as close as possible to the object to be lifted, bending your legs, while holding the object securely, ideally by the handles.
- Keep your back and arm straight throughout the lift, slowly straightening your legs to lift the object in a steady movement and avoiding any jerking.
- Take small movements with your feet when walking, especially around corners.
- Avoid lifting any object that requires you to bend or twist during the movement, for example luggage on conveyor belts. If carrying numerous bags, spread the weight to each side evenly to balance out the strain.

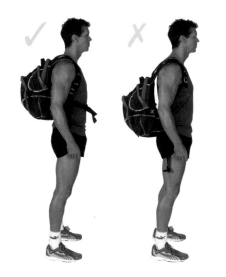

how to carry

Wearing a backpack incorrectly places tremendous strain on the lower back.

- Keep heavy objects close to your body at shoulder height, with your lighter items at the bottom and away from your body.
- Small backpacks should be worn high and snug to the upper back/shoulder area, with front straps pulled tight and any frontal straps used to prevent movement while walking.
- Larger backpacks ideally will have a hip belt, which you should tighten before the shoulder straps to help distribute the weight predominantly onto the hips.

how to sit

- Choose a chair that contours to your spine (especially the lower back), with dense material able to support your weight evenly.
- Seat cushions need to be sloping at the front, with your legs not in contact with the chair and feet flat on the floor to improve circulation.
- Arm rests reduce the strain on your shoulders, neck, and back.
- Your seated position should enable you to keep your spine upright, with your elbows close to your sides, buttocks touching the rear of the chair, and your knees even or slightly higher than your hips.
- Avoid slouching, leaning to your side, crossing your legs while upright, and sitting stationary for long periods.
- Breathable fabric, castors, height adjusters, and swivel legs are all beneficial.

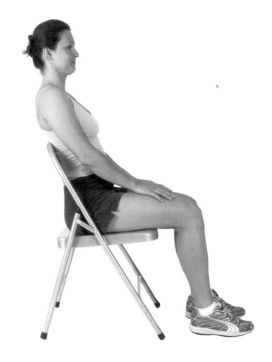

how to stand

- Be aware of your standing position, stand tall, and avoid slouching, keeping your joints in correct alignment so that muscles are worked properly.
- Aim to keep your head up, with your earlobes in line with the middle of your shoulders.
- Shoulder blades should be back, with chest forward, stomach in, and legs straight.
- Keep feet firmly on the floor and facing forward, shoulder width apart.
- Avoid standing in the same position for long periods.

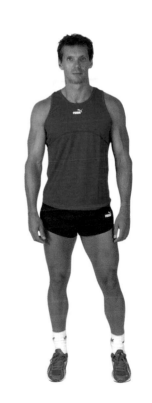

general labor

General laboring can range from construction work to gardening, cleaning the house, or ironing the clothes. These activities are not often associated as forms of exercise, so many people will have no inclination to stretch for what can actually be a long aerobic and muscular workout.

If time is not a problem, perform the mobility exercises on pages 16–19, followed by the dynamic movements on pages 130–149. You will soon find that once you know the movements, you can combine them and reduce the time spent.

Whatever tasks you're performing, it's essential to make sure the tools you're using are not only designed for that job, but are also suited to you. Digging a hole is hard enough, and having the wrong shovel—perhaps the handle is too short or the head is too big—will add unnecessary effort to the job.

Look at varying your working position in order to work different muscles, and thus enable those that have been working to have a rest. Simply changing hands while cleaning or ironing will help prevent shoulder and wrist tension.

Stopping to stretch or mobilize the joints throughout your manual work should be encouraged wherever possible. Avoid stretching when you feel sore—the simple key is to stretch to keep this soreness from occurring. If soreness does occur, then relieve the tension first with the mobility exercises and then use the stretches related to the area of pain.

Having a warm bath at the end of the day will help relax your muscles. Do the cool-down stretches on page 151 after your bath to help reduce muscle soreness and prevent long-term muscular or joint injuries.

Perform the quick stretch routine on pages 176–177 before you begin the stretches opposite.

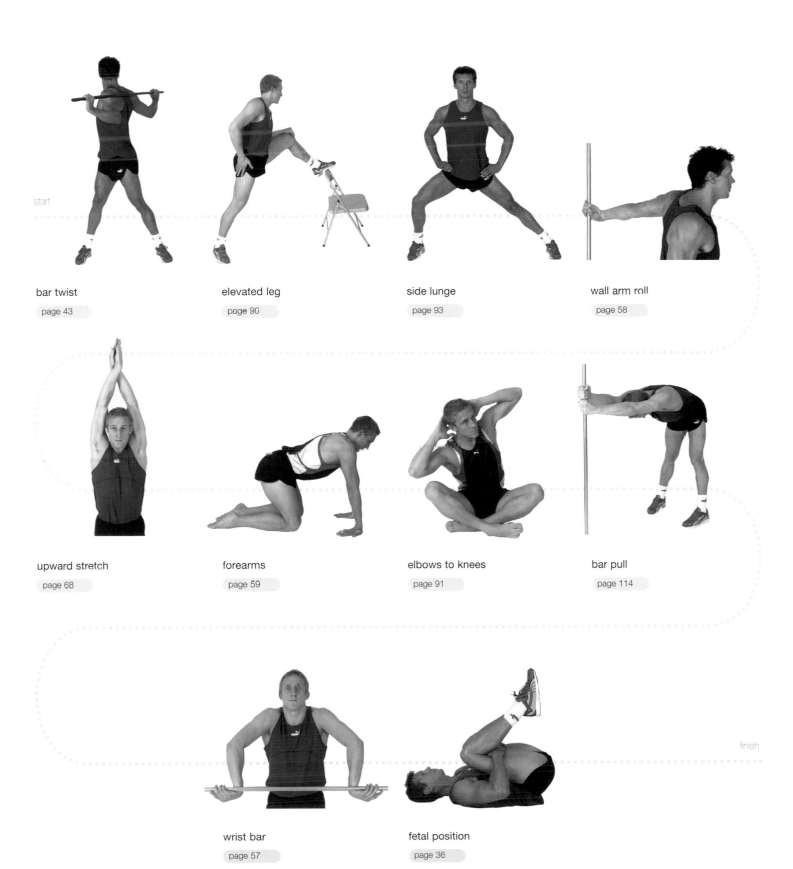

start

bar twist

page 43

elevated leg

page 90

side lunge

page 93

wall arm roll

page 58

upward stretch

page 68

forearms

page 59

elbows to knees

page 91

bar pull

page 114

finish

wrist bar

page 57

fetal position

page 36

office stretch

For anyone who works constantly at a desk, having regular short breaks to simply stretch the legs will greatly reduce the stress that is placed on the back while in a compressed position. The back is not the only area to suffer; repetitive strain injuries (RSI) are injuries involving damage to muscles and tendons and are most commonly associated with keyboard operators, affecting their hands, wrists, and elbows.

Normal muscular injuries occur due to overexertion or trauma, RSIs are caused over a period of time, as the muscles and tendons gradually become tensed up and damaged.

Try to eliminate the causes of discomfort at work—these could be incorrect desk setup, insufficient rest time, poorly designed keyboard and mouse, and so on.

Stretching in the office does not require you to get changed into your gym clothing. Even while stuck at your desk you can perform all of the mobility exercises on pages 16–19. Work on the mobility exercises throughout the day and use any short breaks to perform the dynamic stretches on pages 130–149 in a slow, controlled motion.

Being forced to stretch the muscles in a cold state requires the muscles to be stretched gradually. Hold these stretches for a few seconds only, before relaxing the muscle and repeating the stretch another four to five times, gradually increasing the length of time you hold it. Breathe comfortably throughout this process, inhaling as you begin the stretch and exhaling as you relax.

Prevention is the simple key to avoiding muscular soreness in the office. Use your time on the phone, by the photocopier, even sitting in your chair to perform your stretches.

Performing the warm-up stretches on page 151 prior to going to work will help prepare you for the day. Likewise, using the cool-down stretches on page 151 when you return home will ease the day's tension.

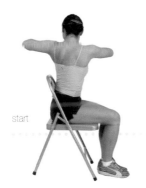

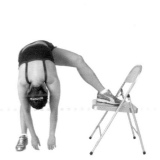

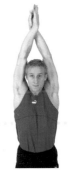

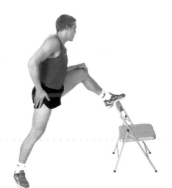

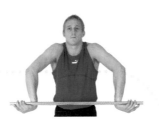

start

trunk twist

page 44

chair slump

page 89

elevated leg

page 96

upward stretch

page 68

wrist bar

page 57

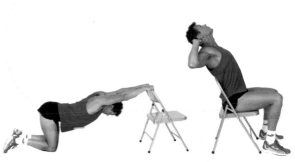

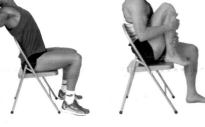

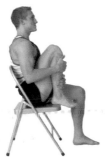

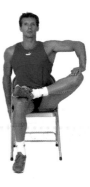

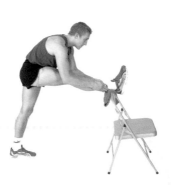

pull and push

page 37

seated back extension

page 76

knee to chest

page 84

seated glutes

page 82

one leg raised

page 126

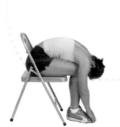

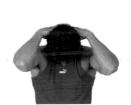

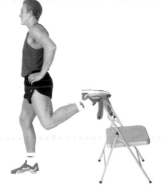

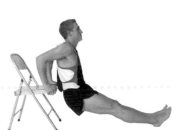

finish

seated toe grab

page 38

chin to chest

page 53

one leg elevated rear

page 104

triceps dip

page 61

traveling

Many of us have experienced the discomfort of being cramped up while traveling, whether it is in the air, on a train, or in your own car. These discomforts can lead to a more serious condition, DVT (deep vein thrombosis), especially for those who have blood clots, smokers, people over forty, those with circulation problems or have recently undergone surgery, and for women who are or have been recently pregnant or are taking birth control pills or hormone replacement therapy.

The main problem areas are the calves, buttocks, and hamstrings, especially during long flights. Fortunately, most passengers should be able to stretch and exercise during the journey. Those that are behind the wheel should plan to stop in a safe area at least once an hour to have a quick stretch, using either the quick stretch routine on pages 176–177 or the dynamic movements for the lower body on pages 130–149. Key points to make your journey more comfortable:

• During your journey, sit comfortably or, if forced to stand, lean against something to reduce the weight on your feet.

• Do the mobility exercises on pages 16–19. Work on all areas that you can mobilize safely. It's important to remember that working your upper body will help circulate blood in your lower body.

• Avoid alcohol and caffeine, as these will dehydrate you—drink water or fruit juice instead.

• Lift and lower your heels, pressing the balls of your feet down against the floor, and then lifting your toes up off the floor. Repeat each movement twenty times or more at least every hour to ease calf strain.

• Straightening and bending the legs, and also bringing your knee into your chest while in a seated position, will help stretch the hamstring muscles.

• Repeated crossing of the legs (knee over opposite knee), alternately five times each leg, will reduce built-up tension in your buttocks, especially if you can increase the stretch by pulling with your arms.

• Wear loose, comfortable, nonrestrictive clothing and comfortable footwear. Elastic stockings, which are widely available from drug stores, can help reduce the risk of DVT in those who are more vulnerable.

• Take advantage of any available time to walk around and stretch.

Stretching before and after your journey will help prevent muscle soreness—use the warm-up and cool-down stretches on page 151. At the end of your journey or during travel breaks, spend a few moments walking, prior to stretching, in order to work any tension out of the muscles.

start

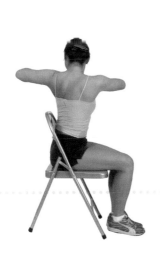

trunk twist seated

page 44

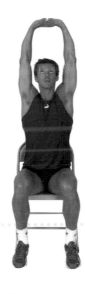

hands interlocked over head

page 57

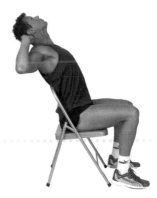

seated back extension

page 76

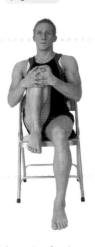

knee to chest

page 84

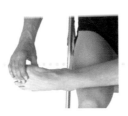

toe pull down

page 109

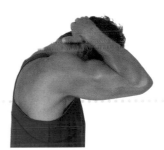

chin to chest

page 52

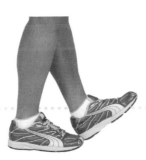

foot and heel raises

page 148

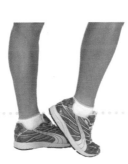

foot and heel raises

page 148

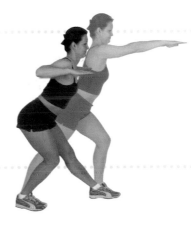

calves and arms

page 134

finish

cool-down stretches

relax/cool-down/breathing

Daily stresses and tension are often built up throughout the day, resulting in muscular tension, especially in the areas of the back, neck, and shoulders; nervous tension; upset stomach; restlessness; irritation; walking or talking faster; excessive smoking, drinking, and eating; crying; and lack of energy. There are many stresses in our lives, but preparing yourself and noticing the signs of stress prior to tense situations will help you cope both during and afterward.

Spend time relaxing each day. It only takes a few minutes to release the tension and stress that can be built up so easily in today's hectic lifestyles. Listening to soothing music in a warm room will prove beneficial.

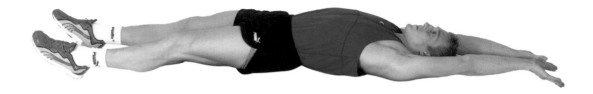

relax stretch A

Lie on your back, making yourself as long as possible by straightening your arms and pointing your toes away from you. Take five deep breaths through your nose and slowly exhale out, increasing the stretch throughout your body. As you inhale, relax totally from the stretch, filling your lungs with air.

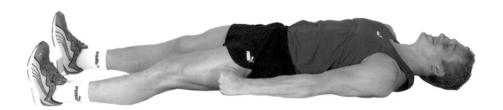

relax stretch B

Lie on your back with hands by your side. Inhale slowly and tense all the muscles up in your body, starting with your feet, working up toward your facial muscles.
Feel and hold the tension in each muscle, then totally relax and exhale deeply before repeating two to three more times. Avoid excessive tensing if you suffer from high blood pressure.

stretch resources

Relax Into Stretch: Instant Flexibility Through Mastering Muscle Tension
Pavel Tsatsouline
Dragon Door Publications, 2001
An illustrated guide to the thirty-six most effective techniques for increased flexibility.

Beyond Stretching: Russian Flexibility Breakthroughs
Pavel Tsatsouline
Dragon Door Publications, 1998
A must-read for athletes. Shows new ways to progress and improve flexibility.

Stretching: 20th Anniversary (Stretching, 20th Ed.)
Bob Anderson
Shelter Publications, 2000
An easy-to-use book on stretching for all age groups and fitness levels.

The Whartons' Stretch Book: Featuring the Breakthrough Method of Active-Isolated Stretching
Jim Wharton, Phil Wharton
Times Books, 1996
New approach to increased flexibility with effective exercises.

Stretch and Strengthen
Judith B. Alter
Mariner Books, 1992
Fully illustrated exercises based on exercise philosophy, for both beginners and professional athletes.

Stretching for Fitness, Health and Performance: The Complete Handbook for All Ages and Fitness Levels
Christopher A. Oswald, Stanley N. Basco
Sterling Publications, 1998
A comprehensive manual with detailed, user-friendly exercises and photos.

Stretch and Strengthen for Rehabilitation and Development
Bob Anderson, Donald G. Bornell
Stretching, 1984
Useful book for those easing into fitness after surgery or injury.

Sport Stretch
Michael J. Alter
Human Kinetics, 1998
Stretching routines for all abilities, combining scientific fact with practical advice.

Stretching Scientifically: A Guide to Flexibility Training
Thomas Kurz
Stadion Publishing Co., 1998
New and unique ideas applied to old established methods of flexibility development.

Super Joints: Russian Longevity Secrets for Pain-Free Movement, Maximum Mobility, and Flexible Strength
Pavel Tsatsouline
Dragon Door Publications, 2001
Expert advice on how to maintain peak joint health.

Complete Stretching: A New Exercise Program for Health and Vitality
Maxine Tobias, John Patrick Sullivan
Knopf, 1992
Clear and easy to follow, with full-color illustrations on every page.

The Complete Idiot's Guide to Healthy Stretching
Chris Verna, Steve Hosid, John Smoltz
Alpha Books, 1998
Exercises for every part of the body to increase flexibility and reduce risk of injury.

stretch websites

www.netfit.co.uk
Stretching tips with a selection of stretches to try.

www.mayoclinic.com
Helpful medical and practical advice on stretching.

www.marathontraining.com
General stretching advice and its benefits and importance for runners.

www.howtostretch.com
Detailed instructions on how to stretch your body, with accompanying photos.

www.sportsinjurybulletin.com
Stretching and flexibility tips to help avoid sports injury and radically improve athletic performance.

www.wholefitness.com
Some simple stretching suggestions for warming up, cooling down, and relieving stress.

www.webhealthcentre.com
Safe guide to stretching exercises.

www.key2fitness.com
Twenty-one stretching exercises, with diagrams.

www.fitness-training.net
Detailed discussion of stretching techniques and flexibility.

www.sport-fitness-advisor.com
Sport-specific training information on stretching for health and sports.

index